# Vital Notes for Nurses:
# Principles of Care

**Vital Notes for Nurses**

*Vital Notes for Nurses* are indispensable guides for student nurses taking the pre-registration programme in all branches of nursing.

These concise, accessible books assume no prior knowledge. Each book in the series clearly presents the essential facts in context in a user-friendly format and provides students and qualified nurses with a thorough understanding of the core topics which inform professional practice.

**Published**

*Vital Notes for Nurses: Psychology*
Sue Barker
ISBN: 978-1-4051-5520-5

*Vital Notes for Nurses: Accountability*
Helen Caulfield
ISBN: 978-1-4051-2279-5

*Vital Notes for Nurses: Health Assessment*
Edited by Anna Crouch and Clency Meurier
ISBN: 978-1-4051-1458-5

*Vital Notes for Nurses: Professional Development, Reflection and Decision-making*
Melanie Jasper
ISBN: 978-1-4051-3261-9

*Vital Notes for Nurses: Principles of Care*
Hilary Lloyd, Helen Hancock and Steve Campbell
ISBN: 978-1-4051-4598-5

*Vital Notes for Nurses: Nursing Theory*
Hugh McKenna and Oliver Slevin
ISBN: 978-1-4051-3702-7

*Vital Notes for Nurses: Research for Evidence-Based Practice*
Robert Newell and Philip Burnard
ISBN: 978-1-4051-2562-9

*Vital Notes for Nurses: Promoting Health*
Edited by Jane Wills
ISBN: 978-1-4051-3999-1

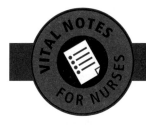

**VITAL NOTES** FOR NURSES

# Principles of Care

## Hilary Lloyd

RN, BSc(Hons), LPE, MSc
Principal Lecturer in Nursing, Practice Development and Research, Deputy
Head of Nursing Research and Development
Nursing Practice Research Centre, City Hospitals Sunderland
NHS Foundation Trust and Northumbria University

## Helen Hancock

RN, BN, MSc, PhD
Post-Doctoral Research Fellow
Centre for Integrated Health Care Research, Wolfson Research Institute,
School for Health, Durham University

## Steve Campbell

RN, RSCN, RHV, BNurs, PhD
Professor of Nursing Practice, Head of Research and Development and
Head of Nursing Research and Development
Nursing Practice Research Centre, City Hospitals Sunderland NHS Foundation
Trust and Northumbria University

**Blackwell**
Publishing

© 2007 by Hilary Lloyd, Helen Hancock and Steve Campbell

Blackwell Publishing editorial offices:
Blackwell Publishing Ltd, 9600 Garsington Road, Oxford OX4 2DQ, UK
Tel: +44 (0)1865 776868
Blackwell Publishing Inc., 350 Main Street, Malden, MA 02148-5020, USA
Tel: +1 781 388 8250
Blackwell Publishing Asia Pty Ltd, 550 Swanston Street, Carlton, Victoria
3053, Australia
Tel: +61 (0)3 8359 1011

First published 2007 by Blackwell Publishing Ltd

ISBN: 978-1-4051-4598-5

Library of Congress Cataloging-in-Publication Data

Lloyd, Hilary.
    Principles of care / Hilary Lloyd, Helen Hancock, and Steve Campbell.
        p. ; cm. — (Vital notes for nurses)
    Includes bibliographical references.
    ISBN-13: 978-1-4051-4598-5 (pbk. : alk. paper)
    1. Nursing.  I. Hancock, Helen.  II. Campbell, Steven, RGN.
III. Title.  IV. Series.
    [DNLM:  1. Nursing Care. WY 100 L793p 2007]
    RT41.L79 2007
    610.73—dc22

                                                    2006036998

A catalogue record for this title is available from the British Library

Set in 10/12 Palatino
by SNP Best-set Typesetter Ltd., Hong Kong
Printed and bound in Singapore
by COS Printers Pte Ltd

The publisher's policy is to use permanent paper from mills that operate a
sustainable forestry policy, and which has been manufactured from pulp
processed using acid-free and elementary chlorine-free practices.
Furthermore, the publisher ensures that the text paper and cover board used
have met acceptable environmental accreditation standards.

For further information on Blackwell Publishing, visit our website:
www.blackwellnursing.com

# Contents

# About the authors

**Hilary Lloyd** is Principal Lecturer in Nursing Practice Development and Research and Deputy Head of Nursing R and D; this is a joint post between City Hospitals Sunderland NHS Foundation Trust and Northumbria University. She has had a varied nursing career, working in acute medicine and care of the elderly as well as some time out of the NHS working clinically in prison health care and in the independent sector. Returning to the NHS her work included managing research trials and practice development. Education, research and practice development have been central to her work. She has held Visiting Lecturer and Senior Lecturer posts in Universities delivering on graduate and postgraduate programmes and developing contemporary nursing curriculum. Hilary leads projects improving the delivery of patient care, increasing the knowledge and skills of nurses and influencing the nursing research and development strategy. She is currently studying for a PhD, exploring the psychosocial needs of stroke patients.

**Helen Hancock** is Postdoctoral Research Fellow in the Centre for Integrated Health Care Research, School for Health at Durham University in the UK. Her clinical nursing background is in cardiovascular medicine in intensive and critical care in Australia and in the UK; both in private and government funded health care. Her clinical appointments have included roles as a Clinical Nurse Specialist, Sister: Training and Development, Sister: Clinical and Unit Manager. Research, education, clinical practice and their development have been integral to her career. Helen completed her PhD at Newcastle University, UK, which examined clinicians' decision making in a cardiothoracic intensive care unit. Her research interests include inequalities and inequities of care in cardiovascular medicine, particularly in relation to decision making. She is currently leading a number of research projects in this area and is also involved in postgraduate education in research and evidence-based medicine. Her academic work remains focused on improving the effectiveness and quality of health care.

**Steven Campbell** is Head of Research and Development City Hospitals Sunderland NHS Foundation Trust and Chair of Nursing Practice, School of Health, Community and Education Studies, Northumbria University. He is also the Head of Nursing Research and Development at City Hospitals Sunderland NHS Foundation Trust, where he leads the Nursing Practice Research Centre. His prime interest is in the development and use of academic skills in the practice arena, the notion of the clinical university. Linked to this emphasis he has held a number of joint appointments, one at the University of Southampton, and another as a doctoral research student, on the topic of mouth assessment. His current expertise in service improvement and leadership is complemented by his international reputation in children's nursing research. He was founding editor of the Journal of Child Health Care, now with Sage, and has published in nursing journals for 30 years.

# Preface

Recent and ongoing changes in health care have influenced unprecedented changes in care delivery and provided nursing with the opportunity to develop into domains previously not thought possible. Nursing is a complex and rapidly changing profession that has risen to the challenges and expectations of twenty-first century health care. Changes to health service delivery have included an increasing emphasis on a multidisciplinary approach to care delivery. As part of this, nurses have taken on more of the work traditionally undertaken by doctors and, at the same time, are being encouraged to engage in evidence-based practice. As the extension of nursing practice increases, it is vital that nurses are equipped with an understanding of the principles of care. This will enable them to provide effective, high-quality care, and to meet the changing needs of health care, which includes changes to the needs of the people they care for.

This book provides a comprehensive account of the principles of care and, while particularly relevant to undergraduate and newly qualified nurses, is also relevant to experienced nurses and those returning to nursing. While the book addresses the principles of care in four successive sections: principles of health and illness, principles of the nursing practice, principles of healthcare delivery and principles of professional issues, the chapters within each of these are also complete in themselves. This approach allows for readers to follow the development of information through the book, or to select particular areas of interest. To enable both to get the most out of the book, cross-referencing to other chapters for further information has been included. Wherever possible, the theory and/or literature included in each chapter has been related to clinical nursing practice, so that the reader can more easily relate and apply the information to his/her practice. As a result it is a useful tool for understanding and applying the fundamental principles that underpin the delivery of effective clinical nursing practice.

*Hilary Lloyd, Helen Hancock and Steve Campbell*

# Acknowledgements

Our sincere thanks to our work colleagues and employing organisations: City Hospitals Sunderland, Northumbria and Durham Universities, for your support. We are especially grateful to colleagues who provided information and valuable comments and for secretarial support in finalising the manuscript. Finally, a special thank you to our families, to Adrian, Andrew and Gill, for your patience, support and encouragement.

Section 1

# Principles of Health and Illness

# Concepts of health

## Learning objectives

- Identify models of health and illness, how these have developed over time and how they impact on care delivery.
- Understand the concepts of health and illness and how and why personal definitions of these differ.
- Understand how personal definitions of health and illness influence health-related behaviours.
- Understand the implications of individual definitions of health and illness for assessment, planning, implementation and evaluation of care.

## Introduction

This chapter will introduce the concepts of health and illness and their implications for the provision of nursing care. This will include a discussion of how health and illness have been viewed historically in health care, and how they are viewed today. Models of health and illness, which help to explain differences in peoples' explanations and behaviour about health and illness, will also be explained and discussed.

## Health and illness

Health and illness are central to nursing practice. As Virginia Henderson stated in 1966:

> *The function of the nurse is to assist an individual sick or well in those activities contributing to health, or its recovery, or to a peaceful death that the individual would perform unaided, if the person had the necessary strength, will, or knowledge, and to do this in such a way as to help the person to independence as rapidly as possible* (Henderson, 1966, p. 15).

From this view, nurses are concerned with the maintenance, improvement and/or support of health and the causes and management of illness. It is, therefore, imperative that they have a good understanding of the concepts of health and illness. Without such knowledge, their ability to practise effectively and to meet the needs of individuals will be compromised.

## What is a concept?

There are many variations on the meaning of a 'concept'. Concepts are abstract notions and ideas. Chinn & Jacobs (1983, p. 200) define a concept as: 'A complex mental formulation of an object, property or event that is derived from individual perception and experience'. Meleis (1991, p. 12) defines a concept as: 'A label used to describe a phenomenon or a group of phenomena'. McKenna (1997) explains that concepts are labels, which give meaning, they enable us to categorise, interpret and structure a phenomenon, but they are not the phenomenon itself.

The concepts of health and illness are more complex than they first appear. This is apparent when comparing personal definitions of health and illness with those of others. While many people view health as the absence of disease, others' views may be based on physiological parameters or may reflect their beliefs about quality of life and the model of health they believe in. Adequate understanding about the concepts of health and illness is imperative as both have implications for the assessment, planning, implementation and evaluation of care.

---

**Activity**

Consider the following:

- What is your personal definition of health?
- What is your personal definition of illness?

Ask a friend, colleague and family member to share their definitions:

- Do they differ from your own?
- What might be the implications of these definitions in your role as a nurse?

---

## A definition of health

In 1958, The World Health Organisation (WHO) published the following definition of health: '. . . a state of complete physical, mental and social well being and not merely the absence of disease or infirmity'. This definition met with the criticism that health cannot be defined as a state, but that it must be seen as a process of ongoing adjustment to the changing demands of day-to-day life. In 1984, the WHO revised its definition to reflect these views: 'Health is, therefore, seen as a resource of everyday life, not the object of living: it is a positive concept emphasising social and personal resources as well as physical capabilities'. This definition recognises the multidimensional nature of health, which includes physiological, psychological and behavioural components.

## A definition of illness

Like health, illness includes physiological, psychological and behavioural components. It is important to distinguish between disease and illness. Disease refers to pathological processes that impair normal bodily functioning. Illness is a socially defined concept about a state of health that differs from what is considered as normal in that community (Harding & Taylor, 2002). Beliefs about what is normal may differ between communities, which means that beliefs about illness will also differ. For example, some communities believe that it is normal (and desirable) to gain weight as this indicates affluence and success, while others view this as a health risk that is not considered normal (and that is undesirable). These beliefs can also differ between individuals. For example, some individuals with a particular disease will not consider themselves to be ill, while others who regard themselves as being ill may not necessarily be suffering from a disease.

Again, like health, illness is a complex concept. Lau (1995) highlights this complexity by defining six dimensions of illness:

(1)  Not feeling normal, e.g. 'I don't feel right'.
(2)  Specific symptoms: these may be physiological or psychological.
(3)  Specific illnesses, e.g. cancer, cold, depression.
(4)  Consequences of illness: e.g. 'I can't do what I usually do'.
(5)  Duration of symptoms, i.e. how long the symptoms last.
(6)  Absence of health, i.e. not being healthy (as compared to 'normal' health).

## Personal definitions of health and illness

While there are numerous definitions of health and illness, such as those above, in the literature, these may not reflect the personal definitions. Personal definitions of health vary considerably. They are affected by a number of factors including age, gender, culture, spirituality, social background and emotional state, as well as health beliefs and health behaviours (Pender *et al.*, 2001; Richards *et al.*, 2003; Schoenberg *et al.*, 2003). Eliciting a person's personal definitions and beliefs about health and illness is fundamental to the provision of individualised care. Without these, it is not possible to plan care that will meet his or her needs. For example, aiming for a patient to run a half marathon after an accident may be appropriate for someone whose definition of health includes a high level of fitness, but may not be appropriate for someone whose definition is based on being able to complete renovations in his/her home.

---

**Activity**

Refer back to your definitions of health and illness:

• How do the definitions of health and illness (above) relate to your personal definitions and those of your colleagues and friends?
• What are the main differences between them?
• Consider what might have caused these in light of the different communities you live in or cultures you embrace.

---

## Models of health and illness

Models of health and illness include those factors deemed important in considering health, illness and health care. Despite their implications for health care, which include influences on healthcare professionals' and patients' decisions about health and health care (Wade & Halligan, 2004), models of health and illness are seldom addressed in the health care literature. The two most common models of health and illness – the biomedical model and the biopsychosocial model – are described below.

### The biomedical model of health and illness

The biomedical model, which has dominated health care for the past century, is based on three assumptions (Wade & Halligan, 2004):

• illness has a single underlying cause
• disease (pathology) is always the single cause
• removal of the disease will result in a return to health.

The biomedical model has its origins in Darwin's theory of evolution and the biological identity of humans. It is based on the assumption that the mind and body function independently, and that physiological malfunctioning causes ill health, with medicines and/or medical treatments used to correct the malfunction(s) (Harding & Taylor, 2002). It is a view that is relevant for many disease-based illnesses and is supported by extensive research (see Porter, 1997). The model recognises psychology and other factors, but as consequences of illness, not as causes of illness. In the biomedical model the medical profession is responsible for any treatment, and for an individual's health or illness, although his or her cooperation with these is expected (Wade & Halligan, 2004).

In physical terms, there have been extraordinary gains in health over the past 50 years. For example, life expectancy worldwide increased from 46 years in the 1950s to 65 years in 1995, there has been a substantial decline in infant mortality, the level of childhood immunisation has increased dramatically and access to primary health care, including water and sanitation, continues to improve (WHO, 1998). Despite these improvements, inequalities in health persist and in some cases are increasing (Acheson, 2002; Department of Health, 2002, 2004a, b). These inequalities highlight the need to view health as more than a purely physical or biomedical concept.

**The biopsychosocial model of health and illness**
The biopsychosocial model of health and illness addresses some of the criticisms about the biomedical model. In contrast to the biomedical model, the biopsychosocial model recognises that social and psychological factors, as well as biological factors, influence a person's beliefs and behaviours in relation to health and illness (Engel, 1977). Dr George Engel created the biopsychosocial model in order to provide a basis for understanding and treating disease, taking into account the patient, his/her social context and the impact of illness on that individual from a societal perspective. The biopsychosocial model builds upon the biomedical model. It distinguishes between the pathophysiological processes that cause disease and the patient's perception of his/her health and the factors affecting it. Biological measures are still seen as important, but they represent only one of the defining factors for the diagnosis and management of disease (Suls & Rothman, 2004; Wade & Halligan, 2004). The biopsychosocial model describes psychological and social effects of disease risk, prevention, treatment compliance, morbidity, quality of life and survival (Lutgendorf & Costano, 2003). Box 1.1 lists the areas in which the two models differ.

## Health beliefs and behaviours

Personal beliefs about health and illness are important as they can influence the way individuals respond to health and illness, i.e. their health behaviour (Harding & Taylor, 2002). Health beliefs shape the way individuals behave in response to their experiences of health and illness. Ultimately, this can influence how a patient behaves in response to advice or information about his/her health. An individual's beliefs

> **Box 1.1 Summary of the differences between the biomedical and biopsychosocial models of health and illness.**
>
> - Causes of illness
> - Types of treatment
> - Responsibility for illness and treatment
> - The relationship between health and illness
> - The relationship between mind and body
> - The role of psychology in health and illness

about health and illness can be understood from the following perspectives:

(1) physiological/physical, e.g. level of fitness or energy;
(2) psychological, e.g. feeling happy or energetic;
(3) behavioural, e.g. eating and sleeping well;
(4) future consequences, e.g. I will live longer;
(5) the absence of something, e.g. illness, disease, symptoms.

Health behaviours have played an increasingly important role in health and illness over the past century. For example, the decline of infectious diseases since the 1800s started prior to the development and use of medication, and a number of diseases in the Western world (e.g. lung cancer, heart disease) are the result of health-related behaviours (e.g. smoking, consumption of fast food) that are not found in other parts of the world.

## Models of health behaviour

In order that the basis of health behaviours can be explained, a number of models of health behaviour have been developed. These fall, broadly, into three categories: stage models, cognition models and social cognition models. These models of health-related behaviours are used increasingly to explain the complex interplay of health beliefs that influence an individual's health behaviours. They are helpful in determining the basis for health behaviour and for answering questions such as:

- How do people decide whether or not to exercise regularly?
- What information is most likely to help people give up smoking?

The models provide a framework for healthcare professionals to gain insight into an individual's health beliefs and therefore his or her perspective of health, illness and the behaviour(s) that result. By doing so they provide a means of meeting individual needs, and of targeting health care to this end.

## Stage models

### The transtheoretical model

The transtheoretical model (DiClemente & Prochaska, 1982) describes the process an individual goes through in making a change or changes to his or her health behaviour. The model identifies five stages an individual goes through in this process: pre-contemplation, contemplation, preparation, action and maintenance. Sometimes a sixth stage, relapse, is added. While the emphasis here seems to be on the process of change, the model also emphasises the interaction between health beliefs and behaviours. During the process of change, the individual weighs up his or her beliefs, the time required to make the change, any costs and benefits of the change. Box 1.2 illustrates the stages of behaviour change in the transtheoretical model and uses a smoker as an example to illustrate how changes in beliefs influence behaviour.

## Cognition models

Cognition models examine the predictors of health behaviours. They developed from subjective expected utility theory (Savage, 1954), which suggests that behaviours result from the individual weighing up the possible costs and benefits of a certain behaviour. For example, a decision to wear sunscreen might be based on an individual weighing up the likelihood of getting sunburnt if he/she doesn't wear sunscreen

---

**Box 1.2 The stages of behaviour change in the transtheoretical model.**

(1) *Pre-contemplation*: in this stage the individual has no intention of making a change to his or her behaviour, e.g. 'I am happy being a smoker'.

(2) *Contemplation*: in this stage, the individual is considering a change, e.g. 'Perhaps I should give up smoking'.

(3) *Preparation*: the individual makes small behaviour changes, e.g. 'I will buy lower-tar cigarettes'.

(4) *Action*: the individual actively engages in the new behaviour, e.g. 'I have stopped smoking'.

(5) *Maintenance*: sustaining the change over time, e.g. 'I have stopped smoking for 4 months now'.

(6) *Relapse*: characterised by a return to the original behaviour, e.g. 'I gave up smoking for 3 weeks, but have started again'.

against not getting burnt if he/she does. His or her behaviour will depend on the importance he/she places on not getting burnt. The importance of this to the individual will be determined by his/her health beliefs about the risks of sunburn and skin ageing and cancer, for example.

### The health belief model

The health belief model (Rosenstock, 1974; Becker & Rosenstock, 1987) is probably the most widely known model of health behaviour in health care. In this model, health behaviour is seen as the result of a set of five core beliefs held by the individual. Combined with an individual's demographic particulars, such as age, gender and socio-economic group, these five beliefs can both shape and help to predict an individual's health behaviour. The five core beliefs are listed in Box 1.3. Like Box 1.2, a smoker is used as an example to illustrate possible health beliefs in reaching a decision about his/her smoking behaviour.

Together with an individual's demographic details, these five health beliefs combine to influence health behaviour. In some more recent versions of the health belief model, health motivation, perceived control and self-efficacy are added (Rosenstock et al., 1994). By making health beliefs explicit, the model can help nurses and other healthcare professionals understand the reasons for an individual's health behaviours. Gaining an understanding of the beliefs that inform behaviour provides a way of addressing why, for example, an individual is behaving in a certain way, or appears to be ignoring advice about a health problem. Health beliefs that are based on poor or inaccurate information can have important and detrimental effects on health behaviour and therefore on health. Identifying these provides a way of explaining health behaviours, and is the first step to modifying health behaviours. It is important to remember that not all beliefs have the same impact on health behaviour.

---

### Box 1.3 The five core health beliefs included in the health belief model.

(1) *Susceptibility to illness*, e.g. 'Smoking increases my chances of getting lung cancer'.
(2) *Severity of illness*, e.g. 'Lung cancer is a serious illness'.
(3) *Costs involved in carrying out the behaviour*, e.g. 'Stopping will make me put on weight'.
(4) *Benefits involved in carrying out the behaviour*, e.g. 'Stopping will save me money'.
(5) *Cues to action (may be internal)*, e.g. 'My friend has just been diagnosed with cancer'.

> **Box 1.4 Health beliefs that combine to shape behavioural intentions.**
>
> - *Attitude towards a behaviour*: comprised of both a positive or negative evaluation of the particular behaviour and beliefs about the outcome of the behaviour.
> - *Subjective norm*: comprised of the perception of social norms and pressure to perform a behaviour, and evaluation of whether the individual is motivated to comply with this pressure.
> - *Perceived behavioural control*: comprised of a belief that the individual can carry out a particular behaviour based upon a consideration of internal control factors and external control factors, both of which relate to past behaviour.

## Social cognition models

Social cognition models examine the factors that predict behaviour and/or intended behaviour and, in addition, examine why individuals fail to maintain a behaviour to which they are committed. They developed from social cognitive theory, which was developed by Bandura (1977, 1986).

### The theory of planned behaviour

The theory of planned behaviour (Ajzen, 1985), which developed from the theory of reasoned action (Ajzen & Fishbein, 1980), emphasises intended behaviour as the result of a number of health beliefs. These health beliefs, listed in Box 1.4, combine to shape intended behaviour – referred to as behavioural intentions in the theory.

# Responses to illness or the threat of illness

When considering an individual's health beliefs and behaviours it is often useful to have information about the way he/she copes with illness or the threat of illness, or at least to be prepared for their responses.

## Illness cognitions

Illness cognitions are an individual's implicit beliefs about his/her illness. They provide a framework from which to understand how individuals identify, perceive, cope and behave (Leventhal *et al.*, 1980, 1997). There are five cognitive dimensions of these beliefs; these are listed in Box 1.5.

---

**Box 1.5 Five cognitive dimensions of illness.**

(1) *Identity*: the name of the disease/diagnosis and the symptoms.
(2) *Perceived cause*: may be biological, psychosocial.
(3) *Time line*: how long will it last; acute or chronic.
(4) *Consequences*: limiting consequences, e.g. physical, emotional, financial and those of treatment.
(5) *Curability and controllability*: e.g. cancer versus the flu, control by the individual or by others.

---

The way an individual responds to an illness will be affected, to some extent, by the way he or she interprets these dimensions. For example, an individual who believes that an illness will last only a short time might respond differently to an individual who believes that the illness is long term. Part of a nurse's role is to understand how an individual has interpreted these dimensions. This allows any misguided perceptions to be addressed. As stated previously, health beliefs that are based on poor or inaccurate information can have important and detrimental effects on health behaviour and therefore on health. Chapter 2 will discuss how individuals' beliefs about health can affect their health behaviours.

**Summary**

- While definitions of health and illness can be found in the literature, individual definitions vary substantially and are affected by a number of social, cultural and other factors.
- The two most common models of health and illness are the biomedical model and the biopsychosocial model.
- The view that health is a multidimensional concept and includes physiological, psychological and behavioural components has gained increasing support in recent years.
- Health beliefs shape the way an individual behaves in response to his/her experiences of health and illness.
- It is important for nurses to understand the health beliefs of individuals in their care.
- There are a number of models of health behaviour, which are based on health beliefs. These include: the health belief model, the transtheoretical model and the theory of planned behaviour.
- The way an individual responds to an illness, or the threat of an illness, is also affected by the way he or she interprets the five cognitive dimensions of illness.

# References

Acheson, D (1998) *Independent Inquiry into Inequalities in Health Report – Acheson Inquiry.* Available at http://www.archive.officialdocuments.co.uk/document/doh/ih/ih.htm

Ajzen, I (1985) From Intentions to Actions: A theory of planned behaviour. In: Kulh, J & Beckman, J (eds) *Action Control From Cognition to Behaviour.* Springer, New York. pp. 11–39.

Ajzen, I & Fishbein, M (1980) *Understanding Attitudes and Predicting Social Behaviour.* Prentice Hall, Englewood Cliffs, New Jersey.

Bandura, A (1977) *Social Learning Theory.* Prentice Hall, Englewood Cliffs, New Jersey.

Bandura, A (1986) *Social Foundations of Thought and Action: A Social Cognitive Theory.* Prentice Hall, Englewood Cliffs, New Jersey.

Becker, M H & Rosenstock, I M (1987) Comparing social learning theory and the health belief model. In: Ward, W B (eds) *Advances in Health Education and Promotion.* JAI Press, Greenwich.

Chinn, P L & Jacobs, M K (1983) *Theory and Nursing: A Systematic Approach.* Mosby. St. Louis.

Department of Health (2002) *Tackling Health Inequalities: Summary of the 2002 Cross-Cutting Review.* Available at www.hmtreasury.gov.uk/media//EEDDE/Exec%20sumTackling%20Health.pdf

Department of Health (2004a) *NHS Improvement Plan: Putting People at the Heart of Public Services.* Available at http://www.dh.gov.uk/assetRoot/04/08/45/22/04084522.pdf

Department of Health (2004b) *Tackling Health Inequalities: A Programme for Action.* Available at http://www.dh.gov.uk/assetRoot/04/01/93/62/04019362.pdf

DiClemente, C C & Prochaska, J O (1982) Self-change and therapy change of smoking behaviour: a comparison of processes of change in cessation and maintenance. *Addictive Behaviours* 7: 133–42.

Engel, G (1977) The need for a new medical model: a challenge for biomedicine. *Science* 196 (4286): 129–36.

Harding, G & Taylor, K (2002) Health, illness and seeking health care. *The Pharmaceutical Journal* 269: 526–8.

Henderson, V (1966) *The Nature of Nursing: A Definition and its Implications, Practice, Research and Education.* Macmillan, New York.

Lau, R R (1995) Cognitive representations of health and illness. In: Gochman, D (ed.) *Handbook of Health Behaviour Research*, Vol. 1. Plenum, New York.

Leventhal, H, Meyer, D & Nerenz, D (1980) The common sense representation of illness danger. In: Rachman, S (ed.) *Contributions to Medical Psychology.* Pergamon Press, Oxford. pp. 7–30.

Leventhal, H, Benyamini, Y, Brownlee, S, Diefenbach, S, Leventhal, E A, Patrick-Miller, P & Robitaille, C (1997) Illness perceptions: theoretical foundations. In: Petrie, K J & Weinman, J (eds) *Perceptions of Health and Illness.* Harwood, London. pp. 19–46.

Lutgendorf, S K & Costano, E S (2003) Psychoneuroimmunology and health psychology: an integrative model. *Brain, Behavior, and Immunity* 17: 225–32.

McKenna, H (1997) *Nursing Theory and Models*. Routledge, Abingdon.

Meleis, A I (1991) *Theoretical Nursing: Development and Progress*, 2nd edition. Lippincott, Philadelphia.

Pender, N J, Murdaugh, C L & Parsons, M A (2001) *Health Promotion in Nursing Practice*, 4th edition. Appleton & Lange, Stamford, Connecticut.

Porter, R (1997) *The Greatest Benefit to Mankind. A Medical History of Humanity from Antiquity to the Present.* Harper Collins, London.

Richards, H M, Reid, M E & Watt, G C M (2003) Victim-blaming revisited: a qualitative study of beliefs about illness causation, and responses to chest pain. *Family Practice* 20 (6): 711–16.

Rosenstock, I M (1974) The health belief model and preventative health behaviour. *Health Education Monographs* 2: 354–86.

Rosenstock, I, Strecher, V & Becker, M (1994) The health belief model and HIV risk behaviour change. In: DiClemente, R J & Peterson, J L (eds) *Preventing AIDS: Theories and Methods of Behavioral Interventions*. Plenum Press, New York. pp. 5–24.

Savage, L J (1954) *The Foundations of Statistics*. John Wiley & Sons, New York.

Schoenberg, N E, Peters, J C & Drew, E M (2003) Unravelling the mysteries of timing: women's perceptions about time for treatment for cardiac symptoms. *Social Science and Medicine* 56: 271–84.

Suls, J & Rothman, A (2004) Evolution of the biopsychosocial model: prospects and challenges for health psychology. *Health Psychology* 23 (2): 119–25.

Wade, D T & Halligan, P W (2004) Do biomedical models of illness make for good healthcare systems? *British Medical Journal* 329: 1398–404.

World Health Organisation (1958) *Constitution of the World Health Organisation*, Annex 1. WHO, Geneva.

World Health Organisation (1984) *Report of the Working Group on Conception and Principles of Health Promotion*. WHO, Copenhagen.

World Health Organisation (1998) *The World Health Report 1998. Life in the 21st Century: A Vision For All.* WHO, Geneva.

# Behaviour in health and illness

## Introduction

This chapter will discuss the concept of behaviour in health and illness. It will provide an understanding of these behaviours in relation to the dimensions of psychological and cultural aspects of health. It is intended to provide a level of application to the theoretical models presented in the previous chapter. The importance of holism in nursing is also discussed.

It is important to understand physical, social, psychological, cultural and spiritual factors that may affect the well-being of an individual (Crouch & Meurier, 2005). These factors can affect the way in which individuals respond to health and health care. While the key concepts of health and illness are outlined in Chapter 1, the way in which these relate to everyday nursing practice must be understood in order not only to provide the best care for patients, but also to help patients make effective choices about their health.

## Health behaviour

The ways in which individuals behave in relation to health are influenced by their understanding of health; this is known as their health beliefs. The health belief model is discussed in Chapter 1 as a theoretical concept. It is important for nurses to understand how health beliefs affect the behaviour of every individual in their care. Each patient comes to health services with his/her own set of beliefs and behaviours, and likewise every health professional has his/her own set of beliefs, which also affect their behaviours and attitudes. One of the roles of a nurse is to give health advice. It is often clear what behaviours are needed to prevent disease and lead to a healthy lifestyle, but how often is this advice taken? According to the health belief model, the actual likelihood of an individual changing behaviour to improve his/her health is based on the perceived benefits of the change minus the perceived barriers (or cost) to that change (Payne & Walker, 1996).

There are a whole range of behaviours that patients can exhibit.

---

**Activity**

Can you think of some positive health behaviours that patients might exhibit? These might be behaviours that you would expect of patients. For example:

- seeking help when feeling unwell
- attending hospital following an injury.

Can you think of some negative health behaviours that patients might exhibit? These might be behaviours that you would not expect of patients. For example:

- continuing to smoke when there is clear evidence that it can damage health
- eating unhealthy foods
- not seeking help when injured or unwell.

Can you think of some negative health behaviours that your colleagues or friends might exhibit?

Why do you think people behave in this way?

---

## Illness behaviour

The way in which a person reacts when confronted with a potential illness is known as illness behaviour. Not all individuals react in the same way and this can lead to a variation in accessing health services and also a difference in response to those providing health care. A number of factors influence the way that individuals behave and the actions they choose to take (or not to take). The factors that affect the behaviour of individuals, which will be discussed in this chapter, are psychological and cultural.

## Coping with the consequences of illness

When dealing with death, pain or other consequences of illness, an individual responds in three ways (Moos & Schaefer, 1984):

(1) *Cognitive appraisal*. The individual initially appraises the seriousness and significance of the illness. For example he/she might consider the following: 'Is my cancer serious?', 'How will it affect my life in the long run?'. Knowledge, previous experience and social support may influence the individual's appraisal process. In addition, it is possible to integrate the illness cognitions of Leventhal *et al.* (1980, 1997) (described in Chapter 1) at this stage in the coping process, as such illness beliefs are related to how an illness will be appraised.

(2) *Adaptive tasks*. Following cognitive appraisal, Moos & Schaefer (1984) describe seven adaptive tasks that are used as part of the coping process. These can be divided into three illness tasks and four general tasks.

    (a) *Illness-specific tasks:*
- dealing with pain, incapacitation or other symptoms
- dealing with the hospital environment and special treatments
- developing and maintaining relationships with health professionals.

    (b) *General tasks:*
- preserving reasonable emotional balance
- preserving a satisfactory self-image and a sense of competence/mastery
- sustaining relationships with family and friends
- preparing for an uncertain future.

(3) *Coping skills*. Following cognitive appraisal and the use of adaptive tasks, Moos & Schaefer (1984) describe a series of coping skills that are accessed to deal with illness. These coping skills can be categorised into three forms, which can be combined and vary from event to event.

    (a) *Appraisal focused coping (thinking)*: attempts to understand the illness, a search for meaning. This may take the following forms:
- logical analysis and mental preparation: turning an apparently unmanageable event into a set of manageable ones

- cognitive redefinitions: accepting the reality of the situation and redefining it in a positive and acceptable way
- cognitive avoidance or denial: minimising the seriousness of the illness.

(b) *Problem focused coping (doing):* confronting the problems and reconstructing them as manageable. This may take the following forms:
- seeking information and support: building a knowledge base by accessing any available information
- taking problem-solving action: learning specific procedures and behaviours (e.g. insulin injection)
- identifying rewards: the development and planning of events and goals that can provide short-term satisfaction.

(c) *Emotion focused coping (feeling):* managing emotions and maintaining emotional equilibrium. This may take the following forms:
- affective regulation: efforts to maintain hope when dealing with a stressful situation
- emotional discharge: venting feelings of anger or despair
- resigned acceptance: coming to terms with the inevitable outcome of the illness.

According to Moos & Schaefer (1984), individuals appraise the illness and then use a variety of adaptive tasks and coping skills, which in turn determine the outcome. However, not all individuals respond to illness in the same way, and Moos & Schaefer (1984) argue that the use of these tasks and skills is determined by three groups of factors:

(1) demographic and personal factors, such as age, sex, class, religion
(2) physical and societal/environmental factors, such as the accessibility of social support networks and the acceptability of the physical environment (e.g. hospital can be depressing)
(3) illness-related factors, such as any resulting pain, disfigurement or stigma.

Miller (1992) describes two different coping strategies used by individuals who are facing an illness:

(1) monitors: want to know everything
(2) blunters: adopt avoidance/denial behaviour.

The coping style adopted by an individual will have implications for the provision of information and for ensuring that an individual's decision(s) about his or her health are informed (see Chapter 6 for more information about informed consent).

---

**Activity**

Think about the way you cope with illness or the threat of an illness. Compare this to the ways you have seen patients cope with these.

- How does someone who is a 'monitor' behave?
- How does someone who is a 'blunter' behave?

How could you address the needs of individuals who adopt:

- 'monitoring' as a coping style?
- 'blunting' as a coping style?

---

# Psychological perspectives

Developments in medicine, health and psychology have led to the acceptance that the mind and the body cannot be separated in the way that they once were. The role of psychological factors in the experience of, and response to, health and illness has become increasingly recognised in recent years.

Psychology is the study of behaviour and mental processes (Payne & Walker, 1996). It is an academic discipline that uses theories to understand and explain how and why individuals behave and think as they do. Considering psychological perspectives in relation to health and illness is important for nurses, as it helps them to understand how individuals react in seeking health advice and when they have a health problem.

## *The impact of psychological factors on behaviour*

An example of how psychological factors are important in a patient's treatment is evident in the simple procedure of taking a patient's blood pressure. It is recognised that some patients have a higher blood pressure when they visit the clinic, than they do when they have their blood pressure taken in their home. This is widely known as 'white coat syndrome' or 'white coat hypertension'. Although the title may be misleading, as many doctors no longer wear white coats, the condition is still exhibited in some patients.

The explanation commonly given is that some people experience anxiety during a clinic visit, which leads to a rise in blood pressure. Parati *et al.* (2003) suggest that if blood pressure measurements in the clinical setting are thought to be caused by unusual anxiety, then daytime blood pressure, taken during normal day-to-day activity, should be used as a baseline measurement.

---

**Activity**

Consider a situation where you have a patient coming to see you in a clinic:

- How will you know that the patient is anxious?
- What behaviours might he/she exhibit?
- How will this change your behaviour towards the patient?
- What can you do to help patients with their anxiety?

---

## The dying patient

There is well-documented evidence of how psychological perspectives can play an important part in health behaviours in patients who are dying. Kubler-Ross (1970) interviewed dying clients and outlined five stages a person goes through when facing death. These are denial, anger, bargaining, depression and finally, acceptance. These stages are summarised in Table 2.1. A person's behaviour is very much dependent on the stage that he/she is in.

**Table 2.1** Five stages of bereavement (adapted from Kubler-Ross, 1970).

| Response | Description |
|---|---|
| Denial | Individuals take a position of 'It isn't really happening'. They have thoughts that help them deny the experience. They deceive themselves and others, often convincing themselves that the situation is temporary and everything will return to normal soon |
| Anger | The individual takes a position of 'Why me?' or 'How dare this happen to me?'. The individual often rages with the world for allowing something like this to happen. The individual feels isolated and furious at what is happening and believes it to be unfair. In this stage, outbursts of anger are common in unconnected situations |
| Bargaining | The individual takes a position of 'If I do this, I can make it better'. Such individuals often have feelings of guilt and a responsibility to try to fix the problems. They often attempt to strike bargains, this is commonly with God, or spouses or parents |
| Depression | The individual is passive, taking a position of helplessness: 'This is really going to happen and it's really sad'. At this stage, the individual is absorbed in the intense pain they feel from having their world fall apart. They can be overwhelmed with feelings of helplessness and sadness |
| Acceptance | The individual takes a position of 'It is sad but I have so much to live for and so many to love'. The loss is accepted and the individual concentrates on alternatives to coping with the loss and to minimize the loss |

The five stages – denial, anger, bargaining, depression and acceptance – are a part of a framework; however, it is not a linear process and not all individuals go through these stages or do so in a set order. Grief, as with all health behaviours, is particular to each individual.

### Pain

Pain is another example of how psychological dimensions of health can affect behaviour. Pain is usually considered organic, because of tissue damage, and the treatment is focused around medical treatment. However, there are also psychological dimensions of pain, often referred to as psychogenic pain. This type of pain is experienced in the absence of physical damage and therefore is presumed to be psychological in origin. While both descriptions of pain can be applied to discrete episodes, they can also be manifest at the same time. Pain can be affected by a number of factors, many psychological; these include control, attention seeking, expectations, state of mood and reinforcement of the behaviour patients exhibit when experiencing pain. Horn & Munafó (1997) suggested that if an individual with organic pain is particularly anxious or bored, then the pain can be enhanced. Twycross (1975) observed that the level at which a pain becomes noticeable to somebody, known as the pain threshold, can actually be lowered by using psychological techniques.

## Cultural perspectives

Keesing (1981) refers to culture as shared ideas, rules and meanings. It underpins the way that human beings live and the way they express themselves. According to Leininger (1978):

> *Culture is the learned and transmitted knowledge about a particular culture with its values, beliefs, rules of behaviour and lifestyle practices that guides a designated group in their thinking and actions in patterned ways* (Holland & Hogg, 2001, p. 3).

It is therefore understandable that culture affects people's behaviour in health and illness. Helman (2000) notes that culture has an effect upon people in many ways; these include beliefs, emotions, diet, dress and body image.

### *The impact of cultural factors on behaviour*

Each culture has its own sets of values and norms, and they set the way in which members of that culture communicate with each other, as well as the way they behave. Similarly, all societies have rules/ norms that guide and govern this behaviour by maintenance of the norms. In the case of Western societies, culture defines and regulates various roles and responsibilities, such as those related to friends, family and the workplace (Holland & Hogg, 2001). De Santis (1994) proposed that when patients and nurses meet there are, in fact, three cultures that affect that relationship and subsequent health behaviour of all involved. First, the nurse's own culture and beliefs; secondly, the patient's culture; and thirdly, the culture of the clinical setting, whether ward or health centre.

### Childbirth

Perhaps the clearest example of a health process that is affected by culture is that of childbirth. Even within the different cultures of Western society, attitudes about where to have the baby differ. Most women in the UK have babies in hospital, but there is a growing trend to want childbirth at home. Davis-Floyd (1987) suggests that the behaviour and attitude of the individual towards childbirth depends on whether it is considered to be part of normal life, or a process that requires medical/midwife assistance in hospital. The prevailing culture of the family is likely to have a great influence on the decision of the individual. For midwives and other professionals who assist families in making choices, knowledge of the statistics of perinatal mortality is only one of the many important issues that need to be included in the discussion with the family (Browner, 1996).

### Infant feeding

Culture plays a large part in women's choice of method for feeding their babies. The choice between breast feeding and bottle feeding has been studied and debated since the 1960s. Cultural attitudes lead to prevailing feeding practices. Relationships and discussions with friends and relations (sub-cultures) have a great influence on choice between bottle and breast (Elliott, 1998). Aboud (2002) draws attention to a number of unusual infant feeding practices that exist. For example, before giving breast milk, in some cultures, newborns might be given a spoonful of soft, rancid butter or warm water with sugar to 'oil the pipes and sweeten the vocal cords'. Health visitors and midwives struggle to work out whether they should interfere with such health behaviour if they cannot prove conclusively its direct damage to the health of the baby.

---

### Activity

- Should health professionals encourage breast feeding?
- Do people have established views about breast feeding?
- What are the physiological and social factors about breast feeding that affect the mother and child?
- What are the social and cultural factors that might encourage or discourage breast feeding?
- Are the above any different for the mother's second baby?

# Behaviour and beliefs in health and illness

The health belief model (HBM) places emphasis upon two processes: encouraging people to seek early professional help for signs and symptoms of illness, and improving uptake of health promotion/illness prevention programmes, i.e. immunisations and health screening. The first process involves seeking professional help and is termed a health protective behaviour. This behaviour is seen as a result of the individual's perception about:

- how serious the threat is to his/her health
- cost in relation to benefit
- the link between behaviour and disease
- the society and home
- day-to-day reminders that reinforce the change.

Self-efficacy is the belief in one's own ability to achieve required goals (Schwarzer, 1992). As such, individuals are confident in their own ability, even when other factors might make the achievement of their goals difficult. Individuals' beliefs about the health outcome also depend on what they believe they can actually achieve.

The precaution adoption model (Weinstein, 1988) considers health behaviours as precautionary. There are seven stages to this model:

- Stage 1: Unaware of issue
- Stage 2: Unengaged by issue
- Stage 3: Deciding about action
- Stage 4: Deciding not to act
- Stage 5: Deciding to act
- Stage 6: Acting
- Stage 7: Maintenance

As an example, an individual has heard of the hazard in question, e.g. high cholesterol, believes that others are susceptible, recognises his/her own susceptibility, makes a decision to act, and takes precautions, and would therefore arrange an appointment to have his/her cholesterol checked. Weinstein proposes that some processes are more important at different stages. This is important for nurses in terms of providing information about the actual health risks and then emphasising the personal risk to the patient, which is particularly important in the middle stages of the above model.

The self-regulatory model of Leventhal *et al.* (1997) is a problem-solving model; acknowledging the individual as an active problem solver. There are three stages to the model:

(1) Interpretation of the health threat, this may be as a mental representation of symptoms, messages, cues and possible consequences.

(2)   Developing an action plan or coping strategy, this may be seeking medical attention, self-prescribing, discussing with another or sometimes avoidance, i.e. denial or 'wishing it away'.

(3)   Appraisal, an evaluation of the success of coping strategies or actions, and reflecting on the need for modifications.

In practice, it is important for nurses to understand that these patients' behaviour is as a result of wanting to maintain their health and an attempt to return to the 'normal' state of health. Although this is a positive health behaviour, difficulties occur when the consequences of the condition are that the patient will never return to his/her previous state of health, e.g. severe stroke or amputation. Rotter (1975) has criticised this model as being more relevant to middle-class people, as they are more likely to approach health care in this way.

Understanding health behaviour involves more than knowledge of models; it involves being able to apply skills in healthcare settings and has wider applications, such as in illness prevention, promoting and maintaining health, and working with healthcare systems in reducing illness and its consequences.

## Holism

The implication of the above for nursing practice is the ability of nurses to view the patient as an individual with different health needs, beliefs and behaviours. This is often referred to as a holistic approach. Holism is derived from the Greek word 'holos', meaning 'whole'. Nursing as a profession embraces a holistic approach to care; this is evident in nursing theory and nursing models, which are discussed in detail in Chapter 3.

Helman (2000) emphasises that health-related beliefs and behaviours are affected by many factors. Some of these are linked to the specific culture of each individual, while others are linked to psychological and physical factors. They all affect the behaviours people exhibit in some way. Helman (2000, p. 3) suggests that these factors are:

- nature of the individual (age, gender, intelligence, health experience and state – emotional and physical)
- nature of education (formal and informal, including education that relates to religion or profession)
- nature of socio-economy (social class, employment – or lack of, social support)
- nature of environment (weather, population density, housing, health facilities).

A nurse delivers care in a holistic way when taking in to consideration the physical, psychological and cultural aspects of the individual (Crouch & Meurier, 2005). This is also known as individualised care. More information can be found on individualised nursing in Chapter 5.

### Summary

- Health behaviour is the way in which individuals behave in relation to health.
- The study of psychological related behaviours might help our understanding of how individuals react in seeking health advice and when they have a health problem.
- The study of culturally related behaviours might help our understanding of how culture affects individuals both in seeking health advice and when they have a health problem.
- It is important for nurses to understand how health beliefs affect the behaviour of every individual in their care.
- A holistic approach enables nurses to consider all aspects of the individual.

# References

Aboud, F E (2002) Cultural perspectives on the interactions between nutrition, health, and psychological functioning. In: Lonner, W J, Dinnel, D L, Hayes, S A & Sattler, D N (eds) *Online Readings in Psychology and Culture* (Unit 7, Chapter 2), Center for Cross-Cultural Research, Western Washington University, Bellingham, Washington, USA. Available at http://www.wwu.edu/~culture

Browner, C H (1996) The production of authoritative knowledge in American prenatal knowledge. *Medical Anthropology Quarterly* 10 (2): 141–56.

Crouch, A T & Meurier C (2005) *Vital Notes: Health Assessment.* Blackwell Publishing, Oxford.

Davis-Floyd, R E (1987) The technological model of childbirth. *Journal of American Folklore* 100: 479–95.

De Santis, L (1994) Making anthropology clinically relevant to nursing care. *Journal of Advanced Nursing* 20: 707–15.

Elliott, L (1998) Breast is best? *Health Exchange* 13–14 August.

Helman, C G (2000) *Culture Health and Illness,* 4th edition. Butterworth Heinemann, Oxford.

Holland, K & Hogg, C (2001) *Cultural Awareness in Nursing and Health Care.* Arnold, London.

Horn, S & Munafó, M (1997) *Pain: Theory Research and Intervention.* Open University Press, Buckingham.

Keesing, R M (1981) *Cultural Anthropology: A Contemporary Perspective.* Holt, Rinehart and Winston, Austin, Texas.

Kubler-Ross, E (1970) *On Death and Dying*. Tavistock, London.

Leininger, M M (1978) *Transcultural Concepts, Theories and Practices*. John Wiley & Sons, New York.

Leventhal, H, Meyer, D & Nerenz, D (1980) The common sense representation of illness danger. In: Rachman, S (ed.) *Contributions to Medical Psychology*. Pergamon Press, Oxford. pp. 7–30.

Leventhal, H, Benyamini, Y, Brownlee, S, Diefenbach, S, Leventhal, E A, Patrick-Miller, P & Robitaille, C (1997) Illness perceptions: theoretical foundations. In: Petrie, K J & Weinman, J (eds) *Perceptions of Health and Illness*. Harwood, London.

Miller, S M (1992) Monitoring and blunting in the face of threat: implications for adaptation and health. In: Montada, L, Filipp, S-H & Lerner, M J (eds) *Life Crises and Experiences of Loss in Adulthood*. Erlbaum, Hillsdale, New Jersey. pp. 255–73.

Moos, R H & Schaefer J A (1984) The crisis of physical illness: An overview and conceptual approach. In: Moos, R H (ed.) *Stress and Coping with Physical Illness*, Vol. 2. Plenum, New York. pp. 3–25.

Parati, G, Bilo, G & Mancia, G (2003) White coat effect and white coat hypertension: what do they mean? *Cardiovascular Reviews and Reports* 24 (9): 477–84.

Payne, S & Walker, J (1996) *Psychology for Nurses and the Caring Professions*. Open niversity Press, Buckingham.

Rotter, J (1975) Some problems and misconceptions related to the construct of internal versus external control of reinforcement. *Journal of Consulting and Clinical Psychology* 43: 56–67.

Schwarzer, R (ed.) (1992) *Self-Efficacy: Thought Control of Action*. Hemisphere, Washington.

Twycross, R G (1975) *The Dying Patient*. Christian Medical Fellowship, London.

Weinstein, N D (1988) The precaution adoption process. *Health Psychology* 7: 355–86.

# Nursing theories and nursing models

## Learning objectives

- Understand what is meant by nursing theory, concepts and models.
- Understand the different types of nursing theory.
- Identify key nursing theorists and their models, and be able to summarise their work.
- Understand how nursing theory can be applied to everyday nursing practice.

## Introduction

This chapter will introduce nursing theories and nursing models and discuss how they relate to contemporary nursing practice.

Nursing theories form the basis of professional nursing practice. Basic to any professional discipline is the development of a body of knowledge that can be applied to its practice (Torres, 1990). This knowledge is developed through nursing theory and nursing models. These theories are important as they help nurses to have a better understanding of nursing and they support nursing practice.

Nursing is regarded as an emerging science, it is important therefore for nursing to continue to develop its 'body of knowledge'. This knowledge is usually expressed in terms of concepts and theories.

## What is a concept?

Concepts are abstract notions and ideas. Chinn & Jacobs (1983, p. 200) define a concept as: 'a complex mental formulation of an object, property or event that is derived from individual perception and experience', whereas Meleis (1991, p. 12) defines a concept as: 'a label used to describe a phenomenon or a group of phenomena'.

McKenna (1997) explains that concepts are labels that give meaning, they enable us to categorise, interpret and structure a phenomenon, but they are not the actual phenomenon. Torres (1990) suggests that in nursing the most significant concepts that influence and determine its practice include:

- the human or individual
- society/environment
- health
- nursing.

Broadly speaking these concepts interrelate, and it is these concepts that are essential to both the development of nursing theories and the understanding of them. They are the ideas that together help to formulate the theory.

## What is a theory?

A theory is the result of searching, an exploration for truth. The term 'theory' originated from the Greek word *'theoria'*, meaning 'vision'. There are a number of definitions of a theory.

Powers & Knapp (1995, pp. 170–171) defined theory as: 'a set of statements that tentatively describe, explain, or predict relationships among concepts that have been systematically selected and organised as an abstract representation of some phenomenon', whereas Kerlinger (1986, p. 11) viewed theories as: 'a set of interrelated concepts that give a systematic view of a phenomenon (an observable fact or event) that is explanatory and predictive in nature'.

# Nursing theory

Nursing theories are an organised and systematic expression of a set of statements related to the discipline of nursing. Nursing theory can be thought of in terms of a systematic way of describing, clarifying and exploring an idea in nursing, furthermore, it must both explain and assist nursing practice. A theory should be useful and provide guidance and a theoretical approach to support practice. George (1990) identified the basic characteristics of a theory (Box 3.1).

---

**Box 3.1 The basic characteristics of a theory.**

- Theories can interrelate concepts in such a way as to create a different way of looking at a particular phenomenon.
- Theories must be logical in nature.
- Theories should be relatively simple yet generalisable.
- Theories can be the bases for hypotheses that can be tested.
- Theories continue to assist in increasing the general body of knowledge within the discipline through the research implemented to validate them.
- Theories can be utilised by practitioners to guide and improve their practice.
- Theories must be consistent with other validated theories, laws and principles, but will leave open unanswered questions that need to be investigated.

---

Nursing theories are valuable to nurses at all levels of practice, they influence who nurses are and what they do, and they influence everyday practice. Nurses apply theory to everyday nursing practice in order to describe, inform, determine and recommend nursing practice. A theory identifies, defines and demonstrates the relationships between a number of components. These components include a purpose, concepts, definitions, relationships and assumptions (Torres, 1990).

## Why is nursing theory important?

Nursing theory is very important for a number of reasons. Most importantly, it contributes to the development of knowledge in nursing; it is the basis for nursing science and therefore contributes to nursing being regarded as a science. In addition, it increases knowledge and professionalism in nursing and ensures that practice is based on sound knowledge. It also provides useful and practical tools for practice and therefore enables the delivery of high-quality care.

---

**Activity**

Take a moment and think about the following questions, then write the answers down in your own words:

- What do you understand by the term 'nursing theory'?
- Why is nursing theory important to nursing?
- How does nursing theory influence your professional practice?

---

## *Levels of theory*

There is not only one kind of nursing theory; in fact, there are many nursing theories, which have developed over many years. There are also different types of theory. Merton (1968), a sociologist, identified three classifications of theory: grand theory, which is highly abstract; middle-range theory, which is more focused; and narrow-range theory, also known as practice theory, which is even more specific. In terms of nursing theory, another level – meta-theory – has been introduced (Dickoff & James, 1968).

These theories are classified according to their scope and depth, with levels of abstraction along a continuum from meta-theory, as the most abstract, to practice theories, as the least abstract. This is a hierarchy of theory, with each level influencing the next.

### Meta-theory

This is the fourth level of nursing theory and is the highest level of theory. The prefix 'meta' means 'a change in position', 'after or beyond' or 'on a higher level' (Pearsall, 2002). A nursing meta-theory presents the universal vision of nursing; it focuses on the broad issues related to theory in nursing (Tolley, 1995). Meta-theorists, for example Dickoff & James (1968), purport that theory can exist at different levels of abstraction and that one level of theory cannot be generated until the preceding level has been formulated.

Nursing meta-theory is the most abstract of theories and, consequently, it is not tested easily. Meta-theory has been criticised for being so abstract that it is difficult to apply to practical situations. A nursing meta-theory is actually a nursing theory about nursing theory. McKenna (1997) describes meta-theorists as 'theory watchers'. They do not form theory themselves, but provide meaning and structure to developing theories and act as a critique for the effects of these theories on both research and practice in nursing.

Meta-theory in nursing must be considered as a superstructure, a framework, which is able to provide the opportunity to discover new grand and mid-range theories and models, and to explore how nursing is constructed.

### Grand theory

This is the third level of nursing theory. Grand theories still present a universal viewpoint and have a broad perspective in relation to nursing practice. While they remain diverse in nature, and general as opposed to focused, grand theories are more comprehensive than meta-theories. Fawcett (1993) defined grand theories as broad in scope, less abstract (although composed of general concepts that are still relatively abstract) and having relationships that cannot be tested empirically. Fawcett (1995, pp. 24–25) explains that: 'Grand theories are developed through thoughtful and insightful appraisal of existing ideas or creative intellectual leaps beyond existing knowledge'.

There is some debate as to whether 'grand theory' can be considered an alternative to a conceptual model in nursing (McKenna, 1997). It is estimated that there are over 50 grand theories in nursing (McKenna, 1997). Some examples of nursing grand theories include:

- Martha Rogers' unitary person model
- Margaret Newman's model of health.

In addition, grand theories may provide the foundation for a middle-range theory.

### Middle-range theory
This is the second level of nursing theory. Middle-range theories are less abstract, more comprehensive and more specific. They are limited in scope and have a limited number of variables, which can be tested (Tolley, 1995). Middle-range theory offers a balance; it is sufficiently abstract to explain complex situations, and sufficiently focused to be measurable. According to Merton (1968), middle-range theories have a stronger relationship with research and practice, and this makes them particularly important for practice disciplines. Additionally, Walker & Avant (1995) maintain that middle-range theories balance this level of detail with a level of conceptualisation usually seen in grand theories. As a result, middle-range theories provide nurses with the 'best of both worlds' (McKenna, 1997).

Middle-range theories focus on concepts of interest to nurses and provide knowledge, which is more easily applied to the practice situation. They are concerned with some, but not all, of the phenomena relating to a discipline. Concept analysis is often suggested as a method to develop middle-range theories (Walker & Avant, 1988). These theories explore concepts such as pain, empathy, uncertainty and grief, as well as specific areas of nursing such as prenatal nursing, family care and illness (Chinn & Kramer, 1995). Examples of nursing middle-range theories are:

- Rogers' theory of accelerating change
- Roy's theory of the person as an adaptive system
- King's theory of goal attainment.

The best example of how the different levels of theory relate to each other is Orem's middle-range theory of self-care deficit, which evolved from Orem's grand theory of self-care (Orem, 1985).

### Practice theory

This is the first-level nursing theory. Practice theories are theories that come from clinical practice and their purpose is to explain a specific nursing practice (Meleis, 1991). Practice theories are very specific in their clinical focus, and they are narrower in scope and much more concrete, in comparison to the theories presented earlier. Jacox (1974, p. 10) defined practice theory as: 'A theory that says given this nursing goal (producing some desired change or effect in the patient's condition) these are the actions the nurse must take to meet the goal (produce the change)'.

Practice theory is constructed to focus on a specific nursing problem. The intention is to guide action; in order to do this there must be a goal, a directive for action and a survey list (Dickoff & James, 1968). McKenna (1997) argues that the current emphasis on the development of clinical guidelines to determine best practice in the UK could be construed as the generation of practice theory.

It is important to understand how practice, theory and research are interrelated. In order to practice as professionals, nurses must be able to apply theory. Practice theory is useful in supporting and directing approaches to practice for nurses.

# Nursing models

Nursing models, often referred to as conceptual models, or conceptual frameworks, result in the identification of concepts and assumptions which, when tested by research, lead to the formation of a theory (McKenna, 1997). Models are abstract, providing a general, broader view, whereas theories are definitive, providing a detailed and precise view (Fawcett, 1995). There is much debate about the differences between models and theories. There is some agreement that conceptual models most closely relate to grand theory (McKenna, 1997). Some, however, argue that they are different. Walsh (1998) purports that theories represent a focused approach to explain relationships between concepts; however, models are a set of ideas that provide a framework to guide nursing practice.

With the exception of the work of Florence Nightingale, nursing theory began to develop in the 1950s and 1960s. This has been attributed largely to the development of graduate education for nurses in the USA (Fitzpatrick & Whall, 1989). The search for clarification and explanation in nursing resulted in much debate and questioning, which led in turn to the development of conceptual models of nursing. Some of these models were developed by theorists, for example Hildegard Peplau and Sister Callista Roy, at a time when they were undertaking educational programmes.

---

**Activity**

Take a moment and think about the following questions, then write the answers down in your own words:

- What nursing models do you use, or have you used, in your area of practice?
- How do you think nursing models influence your professional practice?
- How do you think nursing models influence patient care?

---

Nursing models form the basis of nursing practice and are concerned with knowledge about nursing (Walsh, 1998). A number of key nursing theorists and a summary of their models are presented below. There are too many models to present in this short chapter; however, the reader is advised to consult an array of books on this subject for more in-depth information on individual theorists and their models.

# Nursing theorists

## Florence Nightingale

### Definition of nursing

*Nursing is to put the patient in the best condition for nature to act upon him.*

(Nightingale, 1859, p. 133)

### Nursing model

Florence Nightingale's beliefs about nursing form the foundation on which nursing care is still based today. It is well documented that the organisation of nursing into a profession began in the 1800s under her leadership (Torres, 1990). Nightingale considered nursing to be both an art and a science and was explicit in defining nursing as distinct from medicine. She identified the holistic nature of the individual and developed a theoretical focus. This formed the basis for a research tradition in nursing, and was influential in the development of nursing science (Reed & Zurakowski, 1989).

Although Nightingale did not set out a theory for nursing as we would understand it today, her work was influential in developing the first theoretical approach to nursing. Nightingale's major focus was on the environment for the patient. Environment can therefore be considered as one of the core concepts of her work. The principle was that nursing should provide an environment that allowed nature to act on behalf of the patient; this included the provision of ventilation, clean air and water, control of noise, cleanliness and warmth (Torres, 1990).

In her work, Nightingale also identified the concepts of adaptation, need and stress. Although her work has only vaguely defined concepts, it offers a lot in terms of guiding principles and research in its breadth and simplicity.

Many would argue that her work still has relevance today and is the foundation on which all other theories should be viewed. Much of her theory might be viewed as simply 'common sense'; however, within the hospital environment much can be done to reduce stress, improve adaptation and meet patient needs through nursing practice. A clean environment remains a key aspect of practice today.

## Hildegard Peplau

### Definition of nursing

> *Nursing is a significant therapeutic, interpersonal process which functions cooperatively with other human processes that make health possible for individuals.*
>
> (Peplau, 1952, p. 16)

### Nursing model: the interpersonal process

Peplau's theory emphasises the interpersonal nature of nursing and the distinctive contribution that nursing can make to health care (Aggleton & Chalmers, 2000). Peplau developed a theory-based nursing model; she integrated existing theories into her model, particularly those from behavioural sciences (Howk *et al.*, 1998). It is particularly designed for use in psychiatric nursing and concentrates on the use of interpersonal skills and interaction between the nurse and the patient.

This theory recognises that individuals can react in different ways when faced with health-related situations. Peplau emphasises the interpersonal nature of nursing and suggests that there are four phases of the nurse–patient relationship (Aggleton & Chalmers, 2000):

- orientation
- identification
- exploitation
- resolution.

She goes on to describe six key nursing roles, which reflect the interpersonal and therapeutic nature of this theory. These are the role of the stranger, role of resource person, teaching role, leadership role, surrogate role and counselling role, and they relate to the four phases of the theory.

Peplau's model is still of relevance in nursing today and has contributed to the continued development of nursing theory and nursing science. Many aspects of this theory and the nature of the nurse–patient relationship are also integrated into other works; in particular, therapeutic relationships in nursing remain a key focus of current practice.

## Dorothea Orem

### Definition of nursing

*Nursing is meeting the individual's need for self-care action and the provision and management of it on a continuous basis in order to sustain life and health, recover from disease or injury and cope with the effects.*

(Orem, 1985, p. 6)

### Nursing model

Orem developed an approach to nursing theory with a general theory of nursing developed through three interrelated theories:

- self-care deficit
- self-care
- nursing system.

The individual in Orem's view maintains self-care as long as possible, but may require some degree of assistance from others (Johnston, 1989). The focus is primarily on the individual and is based on the assumption that nursing intervention occurs when the individual is unable to meet his/her self-care needs. This intervention continues until (assisted by the nurse) the individual regains independence. Nursing practice involves the activities of assisting, helping and intervening. Nurses intervene in patients' lives to help individuals to maintain well-being, recover from injury or sickness and cope with the effects of illness (Aggleton & Chalmers, 2000).

Orem identified five methods of helping: acting for or doing for another, guiding another, supporting another, providing an environment that promotes personal development in relation to becoming able to meet present and future demands for action, and teaching another (Foster & Janssens, 1990).

This is a highly specific and complex model. It provides a comprehensive model for nursing practice, which promotes the concept of nursing as a profession, and it continues to be utilised as a model today.

It is particularly relevant in such areas as rehabilitation nursing and nursing of long-term conditions.

## Virginia Henderson

### Definition of nursing

*The function of the nurse is to assist an individual sick or well in those activities contributing to health, or its recovery, or to a peaceful death that the individual would perform unaided, if the person had the necessary strength, will, or knowledge, and to do this in such a way as to help the person to independence as rapidly as possible.*

(Henderson, 1966, p. 15)

### Nursing model

Henderson viewed nursing as an independent, unique health profession, which is supported by education, research and collaboration with other health professionals (Runk & Quillin, 1989). Henderson believed that individuals have biological, psychological, social and spiritual components (Aggleton & Chalmers, 2000). Her conceptualisation of health is achievement of independence defined by the individual's ability to function. Independence and dependence (which is caused by ill health) are on a continuum, and it is the nurse's role to assist the individual to regain independence. This is achieved by ensuring that the individual is able to perform the 14 basic needs listed in Box 3.2.

Key to Henderson's theory is the belief that the nurse is an independent practitioner in the delivery of nursing care. She defines nursing in terms of its function; she sees nursing as a deliberate action. The model emphasises providing individualised care, with the nurse and the patient working together in the planning and implementing of care in order to achieve the restoration of health.

Henderson's work has been praised for being uncomplicated and self-explanatory; making it an accessible and understandable guide to practising nurses (Furukawa & Howe, 1990). It has influenced nursing practice and the development of other models and theories of nursing which are commonly used today.

## Roper, Logan & Tierney

### Definition of nursing

*Nursing is helping people to prevent, alleviate, solve or cope with problems (actual or potential) related to the Activities of Living.*

(Roper *et al.*, 1990, p. 37)

---

**Box 3.2 Henderson's fundamental needs.**

(1)  To breathe normally
(2)  To eat and drink adequately
(3)  To eliminate body waste
(4)  To sleep and rest
(5)  To move and maintain desirable postures
(6)  To select suitable clothes – dress and undress
(7)  To maintain body temperature within the normal range
(8)  To keep the body clean and well groomed
(9)  To avoid changes in the environment and avoid injuring others
(10) To communicate with others in expressing emotions, needs, fears and opinions
(11) To worship according to one's faith
(12) To work in such a way that there is a sense of accomplishment
(13) To play or participate in various forms of recreation
(14) To learn, discover or satisfy the curiosity that leads to normal development and health, and use available health facilities

---

**Nursing model**

Roper, Logan & Tierney (1990) identified common nursing requirements shared by all patients. Their model is based on 'activities of daily living'; there are 12 activities identified in the model, which are represented on a continuum ranging from independence to dependence. These are underpinned by Henderson's 14 basic needs; however, they are specifically based on activity and interaction (Tierney, 1998).

The model represents a move away from a disease-based approach to care and describes preventing, comforting and seeking behaviours, which both nurses and patients exhibit in order to facilitate care (Aggleton & Chalmers, 2000). They define the nursing role as preventing, alleviating and coping with problems, and demonstrate a greater awareness of cultural, environmental, political and economic factors affecting health, absent from many of the earlier models.

The model is based on a model for living and suggests that one of the goals of nursing is to ensure minimal disruption to the individual's lifestyle. This model has made a major contribution to nursing, particularly in the UK, being adopted extensively across the acute care setting.

**Summary**

- Nursing science is based on a sound body of knowledge based on research derived from theory. All nurses must be able to apply theoretical knowledge in order to provide high-quality care.
- There are four levels of nursing theory, which range from the highly abstract to the more practical based; all are useful for the development of nursing knowledge, which in turn informs practice.
- There are a number of conceptual models in nursing which have contributed to the way nurses practice.
- Using a model provides a framework for delivery of care.

# References

Aggleton, P & Chalmers, H (2000) *Nursing Models and Nursing Practice,* 2nd edition. Macmillan Press, London.

Chinn, P L & Jacobs, M K (1983) *Theory and Nursing: A Systematic Approach.* Mosby, St. Louis.

Chinn, P L & Kramer, M K (1995) *Theory and Nursing: A Systematic Approach,* 4th edition. Mosby, St. Louis.

Dickoff, J & James, P (1968) A theory of theories: a position paper. *Nursing Research* 20 (6): 499–502.

Fawcett, J (1993) *Analysis and Evaluation of Nursing Theories.* Davis, Philadelphia, USA.

Fawcett, J (1995) *Analysis and Evaluation of Conceptual Models of Nursing,* 3rd edition. Davis, Philadelphia.

Fitzpatrick, J J & Whall, A L (1989) *Conceptual Models in Nursing: Analysis and Application,* 2nd edition. Appleton & Lange, Connecticut.

Foster, P C & Janssens, N P (1990) Dorothea E. Orem. In: George, J B (ed.) *Nursing Theories: The Base for Professional Nursing Practice,* 3rd edition. Appleton & Lange, Norwalk, Connecticut.

Furukawa, C Y & Howe, J K (1990) Virginia Henderson. In: George, J B (ed.) *Nursing Theories: The Base for Professional Nursing Practice,* 3rd edition. Appleton & Lange, Norwalk, Connecticut.

George, J B (1990) *Nursing Theories: The Base for Professional Nursing Practice,* 3rd edition. Appleton & Lange, Norwalk, Connecticut.

Henderson, V (1966) *The Nature of Nursing: A Definition and its Implications, Practice, Research and Education.* Macmillan, New York.

Howk, C, Brophy, G H, Carey, E T, Noll, J, Ramussen, L, Searcy, B & Stark, N L (1998) Hildegard E Peplau: Psychodynamic Nursing. In: Marriner-Tomey, A & Alligood, M R (eds) *Nursing Theorists and their Work,* 4th edition. Mosby, St. Louis.

Jacox, A (1974) Theory construction in nursing: an overview. *Nursing Research* 23: 4–13.

Johnston, R L (1989) Orem's Self Care Model of Nursing. In: Fitzpatrick, J J & Whall, A L (eds) *Conceptual Models in Nursing: Analysis and Application*, 2nd edition. Appleton & Lange, Connecticut.

Kerlinger, F N B (1986) *Foundations of Behavioural Research*, 3rd edition. Rinehart and Winston, New York.

Meleis, A I (1991) *Theoretical Nursing: Development and Progress*, 2nd edition. Lippincott, Philadelphia.

Merton, R K (1968) *Social Theory and Social Structure*. Free Press, New York.

McKenna, H (1997) *Nursing Theory and Models*. Routledge, Abingdon.

Nightingale, F (1859) *Notes on Nursing: What it is, and what it is not*. Harrison, London.

Orem, D (1985) *Nursing: Concepts of Practice*, 3rd edition. McGraw-Hill, New York.

Pearsall, J (2002) *Concise Oxford English Dictionary*. Oxford University Press, Oxford.

Peplau, H E (1952) *Interpersonal Relations in Nursing*. Putnam, New York.

Powers, B A & Knapp, T R (1995) *A Dictionary of Nursing Theory and Research*, 2nd edition. Sage Publications, Thousand Oaks, California.

Reed, P G & Zurakowski, T L (1989) Nightingale revisited: a visionary model for nursing. In: Fitzpatrick, J J & Whall, A L (eds) *Conceptual Models in Nursing: Analysis and Application*, 2nd edition. Appleton & Lange, Connecticut.

Roper, N, Logan, W & Tierney, A (1990) *The Elements of Nursing: A Model for Nursing Based on a Model for Living*, 2nd edition. Churchill Livingstone, Edinburgh.

Runk, J A & Quillin, S I M (1989) Henderson's comprehensive definition of nursing. In: Fitzpatrick, J J & Whall, A L (eds) *Conceptual Models in Nursing: Analysis and Application*. 2nd edition. Appleton & Lange, Connecticut.

Tierney, A J (1998) Nursing Models: extant or extinct. *Journal of Advanced Nursing* 28 (1): 77–85.

Tolley, K A (1995) Theory from practice for practice: is this a reality? *Journal of Advanced Nursing* 21: 184–90.

Torres, G (1990) The place of concepts and theories within nursing. In: George, J B (ed.) *Nursing Theories: The Base for Professional Nursing Practice*, 3rd edition. Appleton & Lange, Norwalk, Connecticut.

Walker, L O & Avant K C (1988) *Strategies for Theory Construction in Nursing*, 2nd edition. Appleton & Lange, Norwalk, Connecticut.

Walker, L O & Avant, K C (1995) *Strategies for Theory Construction in Nursing*, 3rd edition. Appleton & Lange, Norwalk, Connecticut.

Walsh, M (1998) *Models and Critical Pathways in Clinical Nursing: Conceptual Frameworks for Care Planning*, 2nd edition. Ballière Tindall, Bath.

# Principles of the nursing process

**4**

## Learning objectives

- Understand how and why the nursing process developed.
- Understand the five stages of the nursing process and how these apply to clinical practice and the provision of patient care.
- Understand the difference between a nursing and medical diagnosis.
- Understand how nursing theory and the nursing process are similar, how they are different and how they can be used together in the provision of care.

## Introduction

This chapter will discuss the principles of the nursing process and its application to the provision of nursing care. This will include information about the development of the nursing process and the evolution of its present five stages: assessment, nursing diagnosis, planning, implementation and evaluation. It will build on the previous chapter, which discussed the principles of nursing theory, and will discuss the application of nursing theories to the nursing process.

The nursing process, which offers an individualised approach to patient care, was developed in response to dissatisfaction with care, which, at the time, was standardised or protocol driven and did not meet the needs of individual patients. It is not a model or a philosophy, but a way of organising care, and needs to be used with a model of care (Roper *et al.*, 2002).

The nursing process spread throughout the USA in the 1960s and subsequently throughout the UK in the 1970s. In the USA, Bonney & Rothberg (1963) were among the first to call for a more systematic assessment of patients, which focused particularly on their physical, psychosocial and behavioural health. Around the same time, there were moves to develop a three-phase nursing process (Hall, 1955; Johnson, 1959; Orlando, 1961; Weidenbach, 1963). In 1967, Yura & Walsh published a four-stage nursing process, which included assessment, planning, implementation and evaluation. Finally, as a result of the continued development of nursing as a profession, a phase for nursing diagnosis was added (Roy, 1975; Mundinger & Jauron, 1975; Aspinall, 1976), resulting in a five-phase process. The development of the nursing process in the UK is largely attributed to the work of Jean McFarlane, George Castledine and Pat Ashworth who, during the 1970s and 1980s, encouraged the adoption of the nursing process as the systematic approach to the planning of nursing care (McFarlane & Castledine, 1982).

The nursing process offers a problem-solving approach to care. It consists of five phases that are applied in practice through the nursing care plan. The nursing process forms a framework for practice that provides a means of setting outcomes, prescribing actions and evaluating results. While some versions of the nursing process refer to its original four phases, the authors refer here to the five-phase process (Hodgston, 2002). While each phase is considered as a separate step, in practice these five phases take place in sequence. The five stages are: assessment, diagnosis, planning, implementation and evaluation (Figure. 4.1).

# Stages of the nursing process

## Assessment

This first phase of the nursing process involves systematically collecting, organising and analysing information about the patient, and results in the formation of a nursing diagnosis. It aims to answer the question: 'What is the actual or potential problem?' and is usually initiated when there is a discrepancy between the patient's state of health and an optimal state of health. The assessment phase has two parts: information collection and analysis.

### Information collection
In order to inform the management or care of a patient, the information gathered in this phase must include the nurse's assessment of the

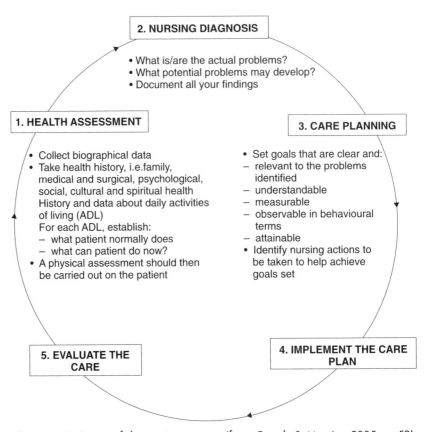

**Figure 4.1** Stages of the nursing process (from Crouch & Meurier, 2005, p. 53). Reprinted with permission of Anna Amugi-Crouch.

patient and the patient's perceptions of him/herself. This information is best gained from the patient (primary source) but can also be gained from other (secondary) sources such as carers, friends and others involved in the care of the patient. These perceptions about a condition or disease are subjective data. In contrast, the data obtained by the nurse are objective. Objective data include physical signs that can be observed and measured. Information can be collected by observation of the patient, through directed conversation and through systematic head-to-toe assessment (Doenges & Moorehouse, 2003). It is important for the nurse to document exact descriptions of what he/she observes, measures and hears. Without an accurate record of this, there is little point in conducting an assessment and formulating a plan of care, as no evaluation of it (discussed later) will be possible. Inherent in such record keeping are the responsibilities of confidentiality (see Chapter 6) and accountability (see Chapter 16) (Roper *et al.*, 2002).

An important feature of the assessment phase is that information is agreed by the nurse and the patient. If the nursing assessment is conducted in consultation with the patient, it is more likely to bring about effective nursing interventions than if the patient is not given the opportunity to participate.

The assessment should include the following (Doenges & Moorehouse, 2003):

(1) A brief statement about the patient's general appearance and behaviour.
(2) A comprehensive health history, including:
    (a) demographic data
    (b) presenting complaint
    (c) history of present illness
    (d) past medical history
    (e) family medical history
    (f) psychosocial history.
(3) Physical examination: explain what you are doing, provide privacy and ask permission before you touch the patient.
    (a) Inspect
    (b) Palpate
    (c) Percuss
    (d) Auscultate

**Information analysis**

Information analysis involves organising the information that has been collected to make it more meaningful and easier to manage. It also reduces the chances of missing important information and allows problems to be prioritised. The analysis also includes identifying the patient's needs, actual and/or potential problems, strengths and/or diagnoses.

---

**Activity**

Think about the last time you carried out an assessment with a patient.

- What types of information did you collect?
- Did you collect both subjective and objective information?
- Can you identify the objective information?
- Can you identify the subjective information?
- Did it include all of the information listed above?
- If not, what was the reason for this?

---

## Nursing diagnosis

A nursing diagnosis is a statement that describes an actual or potential health problem that requires nursing intervention. The introduction of standardised nursing diagnoses came about, in part, as a result of the nursing profession's desire to define the scope of nursing practice, and to standardise the care given by nurses. The formal development of nursing diagnoses began in 1973 with the formation of the National Conference Group for Classification of Nursing Diagnoses in the USA. Nursing diagnoses may be derived deductively, by using a theoretical framework such as Maslow's Hierarchy of Needs for example, or inductively, using patient information collected in the assessment phase of the nursing process (Doenges & Moorehouse, 2003). There are a number of sources of nursing diagnoses worldwide, derived inductively, which include:

- Association for Common European Nursing Diagnoses, Interventions and Outcomes. ACIENDO (http://www.acendio.net/)
- The North American Nursing Diagnosis Association: NANDA (www.nanda.org/)
- The USA-based Clinical Care Classification (CCC) system (http://www.sabacare.com/)
- The Clearinghouse for Nursing Diagnoses, on behalf of the National Conference Group, distributes bibliographies on each diagnostic category, prepared from MEDLINE literature searches.

In addition, there are a large number of published texts that include nursing diagnoses.

The patient's state of health is used to identify his or her nursing care needs. Information is analysed and compared to what is 'normal'. It is important to remember that 'normal' should be considered in relation to what is normal (1) for the general population and (2) for the patient.

The nursing diagnosis may not be a problem. It may be that the patient is in normal health but that he or she may have health-related needs. These may be longer-term needs, such as a lack of knowledge about dietary requirements to be able to maintain normal health, for example. There are a huge number of nursing diagnoses, and one patient may have more than one actual or potential nursing diagnosis relating to the same cause or its consequences. For example, a patient who is immobile as a result of a traumatic injury may be assessed as having a number of nursing diagnoses, including the 'actual impaired skin integrity', 'actual impaired physical mobility', 'potential for post-traumatic stress', 'potential for altered bowel function' and 'potential for impaired skin integrity related to immobility'.

Identifying the cause (aetiology) of the actual or potential problem, as well as the nursing diagnosis, is important, as this informs the type of nursing intervention(s) to be implemented. Nursing interventions may be very different depending on the aetiology. A nursing diagnosis is made on the basis of a collection of information, not just on one observation, clinical sign (scratching, vomiting or sputum), or symptom (itching, pain or nausea). The information needed to make a nursing diagnosis is arranged as shown in Box 4.1 (Doenges & Moorehouse, 2003).

### The difference between nursing and medical diagnoses

Nursing and medical diagnoses differ in that doctors reach a diagnosis on the basis of abnormalities of structure or function, while nurses reach a diagnosis on the basis of the patient's ability to function as a result of (actual or potential) problem(s) caused by the abnormal structure or function. Medical diagnoses have a narrower focus than nursing diagnoses because they are based on pathology. A nursing diagnosis takes into account the psychological, social, spiritual and physiological responses of the client and family (Doenges & Moorehouse, 2003). A doctor, for example, would make a diagnosis of 'stroke' while a nurse

---

**Activity**

Using the information in Box 4.1, identify the 'PES' components of each of these diagnostic statements:

- pyrexia, related to a wound infection, evidenced by inflammation around the wound, elevated temperature, flushed skin, tachycardia and tachypnoea
- acute pain, related to abdominal distension as evidenced by verbal reports, non-verbal communication (guarding and posture), tachycardia and tachypnoea.

Can you think of examples of actual and potential problems for the following patients?

- A 60-year-old lady who has had a hip replacement.
- A 30-year-old man who lost consciousness following a motorbike accident.

Can you think of the nursing diagnoses you might use for the following patients?

- A patient with an elevated temperature:
  (a)   due to an infection of unknown origin
  (b)   due to a thyroid problem.
- A person requiring information about a healthy diet:
  (a)   who is overweight
  (b)   who is undernourished.
- A person with terminal cancer:
  (a)   who is in pain
  (b)   who is anxious.

---

**Box 4.1 Information needed to make a nursing diagnosis (after Doenges & Moorehouse, 2003).**

*P = Problem (actual or potential)*: the key to accurate nursing diagnosis is identification that focuses attention on a current risk or potential physical or behavioural response to health or illness that may interfere with the patient's quality of life. It deals with concerns of the patient (and others) and the nurse that require nursing intervention and management.

*E = Aetiology*: this is the suspected cause or reason for the response that has been identified from the assessment. The nurse makes inferences based on knowledge and expertise, such as understanding of pathophysiology, and situational or developmental factors. One problem or need may have several suspected causes.

*S = Signs and symptoms*: these are the manifestations (or cues) identified in the assessment that substantiate the nursing diagnosis. They are listed as subjective and objective data.

---

would make a diagnosis of 'impaired physical mobility', which has occurred as a result of the stroke. However, there are exceptions to this in the case of emergency situations, where, for example, a nurse, doctor or other healthcare professional may identify a cardiac arrest and initiate appropriate and immediate treatment.

## *Planning*

Once information about the patient has been collected and analysed, priorities for care should be identified. This allows the nurse to make a distinction between life-threatening problems, those requiring urgent attention, those requiring less urgent attention and those that will require long-term attention.

The care plan stems directly from the individual patient's problems or nursing diagnoses. It is not a stereotyped treatment plan. It involves an interactive process to ensure continuity of care that will meet the patient's unique needs. Plans include behavioural objectives and desired outcomes, so that it is clear how the desired outcomes will be achieved (Hodgston, 2002). These should include patient goals which are the desired result of nursing care, and nursing orders, which describe what the nurse will do to help the patient achieve these goals. Patient goals should be clear and succinct, observable, measurable, realistic, written with a specific time frame and agreed by the nurse and the patient (Doenges & Moorehouse, 2003).

---

> **Activity**
>
> - Using a nursing diagnosis you have used recently, formulate a plan of care, including a time frame for that patient.
> - Assuming this is a real plan of care, think about whether or not you will include the patient in formulating the plan and how this might change the plan.

## Implementation

This fourth phase transforms the plan of care into action. Professionals other than the nurse will be implementing the care plan, so it is important that all parts of the plan are detailed enough to enable it to be implemented effectively. During this phase the nurse should reassess the patient and ensure that the care plan is accurate and appropriate, carry out the orders and record any action or intervention (Doenges & Moorehouse, 2003).

> **Activity**
>
> Think about a care plan that you have formulated, or that you have been involved in implementing, and about how effectively the care plan was implemented.
>
> - What worked well and why?
> - Were your colleagues able to implement the plan of care in your absence?
> - Is there anything that you would change next time?

## Evaluation

This final phase of the nursing process involves comparing the outcomes of the care plan with its objectives. The patient's health status is compared to that described in the objectives, to determine whether these were achieved (Hodgston, 2002). This results in one of the following:

- objectives successfully achieved
- objectives partially achieved
- objectives not achieved.

If any objectives were not achieved, as well as identifying ways to achieve these, there is a need to assess why not and to review the nursing process. This may be done in a number of ways:

- revise the objectives
- identify and implement other actions
- collect and analyse more information about the patient and review the nursing diagnoses on the basis of this.

This process describes a return to the assessment phase of the nursing process and highlights its cyclical nature. Often, because of the changing needs of the patient, the process is repeated a number of times before objectives of care are achieved (Hodgston, 2002).

---

**Activity**

Think about the nursing process and the evaluation of care that has been provided.

- Does evaluation take place regularly?
- Who is responsible for evaluating care?
- Why is evaluation important?

---

# The nursing process and nursing models

It is important to distinguish between the nursing process – a systematic approach to care – and models of nursing. Nursing models have emerged from the human sciences. Generally, they describe what nursing is, or what it should be, with the aim of helping nurses, and others, to understand more fully what they are doing and why. Many describe the essential components of nursing practice, the theoretical basis of these and the values required for their application in practice as well as suggesting practical approaches to care (Torres, 1990). The nursing process is not a model of nursing, but a series of steps that can be used in planning and delivering care. While it is not possible to consider all nursing theorists, the following discussion shows how some nursing theorists viewed the nursing process (for more information on nursing models refer to Chapter 3). Due to the recent addition of nursing diagnosis to the nursing process, this phase is not addressed in the nursing models presented.

## *Hildegard Peplau*

Peplau's (1969) continuum of the four phases – orientation, identification, exploitation and resolution – can be compared to the nursing process. Both are sequential and focus on therapeutic interactions. Both use problem-solving techniques for the nurse and patient to collaborate on, with the aim of meeting the patient's needs. Both go from general to specific and both include observation, communication and recording as tools used by nursing. According to Peplau, nursing functions also include the clarification of information given by the doctor to the patient as well as gathering other information that may indicate other problems. While the nursing process takes the total environment into account and views the patient more collectively as a group, family or community, Peplau (1969) focuses on a specific nurse–patient relationship.

When referring to Peplau's theory, it is important to remember that it was first published in 1952 and that changes to nursing roles since then mean that today's nurse has increasing responsibility for patient management that may or may not be provided by a doctor (George, 1990). Similarly, the variables of the nursing situation, such as needs, frustration, conflict and anxiety, referred to by Peplau have been replaced by family dynamics, socio-economic constraints and so on. There is also a greater emphasis placed on patients achieving a fuller health potential through health promotion and health maintenance.

## Assessment

Peplau does not use the term 'assessment' in her theory, but refers to an orientation phase, which parallels the beginning of the assessment phase in the nursing process. Both the nurse and patient come together and work through the recognition, clarification and definition of the factors related to a need(s) of the patient. While there are similarities between the assessment phase of the nursing process and Peplau's orientation phase, the relationship between the nurse and the patient appear more equal in orientation than in assessment. There is an emphasis on developing mutual regard and trust that should ease any patient tension or anxiety. The orientation phase is an important part in building the patient's sense of security (Aggleton & Chalmers, 2000). Unlike the nursing process, in which data collection occurs during the nursing assessment and reassessment, data collection is continuous throughout Peplau's four phases (George, 1990).

## Planning

During the identification phase the patient begins to identify the nurse as someone who can help. During this phase a nursing diagnosis will be made and a care plan formulated. Patients are involved in the identification of goals, for which they provide the information that the nurse needs in order to identify what these should be (Peplau, 1969).

## Implementation

Peplau has little to say about the specific interventions nurses make during this phase. Instead, she places emphasis on the nurse using all means at her disposal to alleviate tensions and anxiety, to remove blocks to further development and to aid personal and interpersonal growth. The nurse may provide access to resources, may counsel and may take the role of others in order to help the patient develop a better insight into the problems that are being experienced. What Peplau (1969) referred to as professional closeness is an essential part of the nurse–patient relationship at this stage in its development, but through the exploitation phase, it is the prime responsibility of the patient to move forward. The difference between Peplau's model and that of most others is that the patient must carry out the chief actions in this phase. The nursing role is one of encouragement and of supplying necessary resources to the patient.

### Evaluation

Peplau refers to the resolution phase, which occurs toward the end of the nurse's relationship with the patient. Here the patient ceases to identify with the nurse and the nurse also withdraws from the relationship to reflect on what has been achieved. In Peplau's (1969) model, resolution can only occur when the patient is able to be free from nursing assistance and is able to act independently. The completion of the resolution phase is one measure of the success of the activities undertaken during all the other phases.

## Dorothea Orem

Orem's (1959) self-care model emphasises the existence of biological, psychological and social systems within the person. According to Orem, a person is a functional, integrated whole with a motivation to achieve self-care.

### Assessment

Orem (1959) rarely uses the term 'assessment'. Instead she refers to nurses undertaking an 'investigative operation' or nursing history to determine whether or not a self-care deficit is present, and to arrive at a nursing diagnosis. She suggests that, by taking five types of information from the patient, nurses will be able to make decisions about the planning and implementation of care. These five types of information are:

(1)  those demands being made on the individual for self-care
(2)  the individual's ability to meet these demands
(3)  if a self-care deficit is found, the nurse must establish a reason for it
(4)  whether the individual's present state allows for safe involvement in self-care
(5)  the patient's potential for re-establishing self-care.

Orem sees assessment as a continuous process, with more information being gathered as the relationship develops between nurse and patient. She also argues for the involvement of the family and significant others in the assessment process.

## Planning

Following the nursing assessment, the nurse and patient embark upon a process of planning. Orem refers to this as the point at which 'prescriptive operations' are made. These specify the care that will be implemented in order to meet therapeutic self-care demand(s) and self-care need(s). The contributions of the nurse and the patient are also agreed (Aggleton & Chalmers, 2000). The nurse should negotiate with the patient whether nursing interventions are to be wholly compensatory, partially compensatory or supportive–educative. Once the nurse has identified reasons for a patient's self-care deficit(s), goals can be set and interventions planned. Longer-term goals are likely to be the restoration of balance between self-care abilities and self-care needs. The extent to which nursing interventions can take place will depend on the extent to which self-care can be undertaken by patients, their families or significant others (Orem, 1959).

## Implementation

This involves both the patient, and his/her family and the nurse undertaking activities to meet therapeutic self-care demands as well as particular self-care needs. The following ways in which the nurse can assist in implementing a care plan are suggested by Orem (1959):

- doing for or acting for another
- guiding or directing another
- providing physical support
- providing psychological support
- providing an environment supportive of development
- teaching another.

## Evaluation

Evaluation focuses on the extent to which the balance between self-care and self-care demands has been maintained, re-established or improved. Orem's (1959) theory presents a three-step method to determine self-care deficits and to define the roles of the person or nurse to meet self-care demands:

- Step 1: the diagnosis and prescription phase, determining if nursing is needed as well as ongoing assessment of why a person should be under nursing care.
- Step 2: the designing of a system of nursing and planning for its delivery.
- Step 3: the initiation, conduct and control of assisting actions to compensate for the patient's self-care limitations. To overcome, when possible, self-care limitations and foster and protect the patient's self-care abilities. Step 3 includes the production and management of the nursing system and evaluation.

These three steps are considered by Orem (1959) to be the technical components of the nursing process. She emphasises that they must be coordinated with the interpersonal and social processes within nursing situations.

## Virginia Henderson

According to Henderson, nursing care is most usually needed when a person is unable to carry out activities contributing to health, recovery or a peaceful death. Henderson (1960) does not explicitly recommend the use of the nursing process. Rather, she argues that the assessment of a patient's needs should involve negotiation between the nurse and patient.

Henderson (1960) viewed the nursing process as the application of a logical approach to solving a particular problem or problems. The steps she refers to are those of the scientific method. She compares the nursing process to the traditional steps of the medical process as if the language has been changed to fit nursing's purpose. She questions the limited focus of the nursing process on problem solving, and views its focus on a rational approach to nursing as undermining the value of intuition (Henderson, 1960).

### Assessment
*Information collection*
Although Henderson does not refer to assessment, it is implied from her description of the 14 components of basic nursing care. For example, in assessing the first component – breathing – the nurse gathers all relevant data about the patient's respiratory status. This data gathering continues until all components are assessed.

*Analysis*
To complete the assessment the nurse analyses the data. According to Henderson, the nurse must have knowledge of what is normal in health and disease in order to do so. With a scientific knowledge base, the nurse draws conclusions from the assessment with the aim of determining the cause of the patient's unmet need(s), so that goals can be set. Henderson advocates that long-term, intermediate and short-term goals should relate to the causes of problems identified during the assessment.

### Planning
Once the nursing diagnosis has been made, the nurse moves on to the planning phase of the nursing process. While she does not use the same terminology as the nursing process, Henderson uses the same ideas described in the planning phase. Henderson's commitment to the individual independently fulfilling fundamental human needs means

that nurses are. Likely to negotiate short-term, interim term and long-term goals with the patient.

**Implementation**

For Henderson, implementation is based on helping the patient meet the 14 components in such as way that it 'promotes the physician's therapeutic plan'. In doing so she recognises the complementary relationship between nursing and medicine (Aggleton & Chalmers, 1986). However, she is not clear about what care nurses might deliver, and nursing interventions take the form of individualised nursing actions aimed at achieving unique agreed goals. Three types of nurse–patient relationship, each with its own type of intervention, are identified (Aggleton & Chalmers, 2000):

(1)   the nurse can act as a substitute for the patient;
(2)   he or she can act as helper; or
(3)   he or she can act as assistant.

**Evaluation**

Evaluation occurs through an examination of the extent to which, following an intervention, the patient has been helped to meet his or her fundamental needs (Henderson, 1960).

## *Roper, Logan & Tierney*

The Roper, Logan & Tierney model (Roper *et al.*, 1980) was first published under the title *The Elements of Nursing*. The model identified 12 activities of living, the key factors that affect them, and four components of the nursing process (assessing, planning, implementing and evaluating).

In their model, four of its components: the lifespan, activities of daily living, factors influencing activities of daily living and the dependence/independence continuum, underpin the fifth component: individualising nursing. This is framed by the nursing process, conceptualised in the model as a cyclical process, moving more or less rapidly through its four stages, depending on circumstances (Tierney, 1998). Roper *et al.* (2002) stress that the four phases (assessment, planning, implementation and evaluation) are interactive, and that this is important because it means that the process is dynamic and includes continuous feedback.

**Assessment**

Roper *et al.*'s (1980) activities of daily living provide a good framework for the assessment phase of the nursing process. This not only includes an assessment of the individual's ability to carry out the activities of daily living themselves, but also includes the individual's views and beliefs about this, and has the potential to increase understanding about the factors that influence the individual. Roper *et al.* (1980) stress the importance of viewing assessment not as a one-off activity, but that it should be an ongoing activity, which includes: collecting information from or about the person, reviewing the collected information, identifying the person's problems with activities of daily living and identifying priorities among the problems (Roper *et al.*, 2002). They state that the assessment should include biographical and health data, activities of daily living, and the individual's problems.

### Planning

For Roper *et al.* (2002), the objective of this stage is to:

- prevent identified potential problems with any of the activities of daily living from becoming actual ones
- to solve identified actual problems
- where possible, to alleviate those that cannot be solved
- to help the person cope positively with those problems that cannot be alleviated or solved
- to prevent recurrence of a treated problem
- to help the person to be as comfortable and pain free as possible when death is inevitable.

This should be achieved by setting goals or objectives of care, which are included in a nursing care plan. They argue that because of the collaborative nature of health care, one plan of care, including a nursing care plan related to activities of daily living and from medical or other prescriptions, should be formulated (Roper *et al.*, 2002).

### Implementation

Roper *et al.* (2002) recognise that the tradition of nursing has been associated with 'doing' and that nurses are familiar with the implementation process. They stress the value of making explicit the thinking and decision making that underpins and explains the nursing interventions within this phase. They suggest that supplementary notes might be used to document the rationale for nursing interventions.

### Evaluation

Roper *et al.* (2002) stress the importance of this stage of the nursing process as, for them, it provides a basis for ongoing assessment and planning as the circumstances and problems of the patient change. Essentially, they believe that this stage of the nursing process aims to find out whether or not (or to what extent) the goals that were set have been (or are being) achieved. They suggest that the following questions might be used to evaluate the achievement of each goal:

- Is it partially achieved and is more information needed before reconsidering whether or not to continue or adapt the intervention?

- Is the problem unchanged or static, and should the nursing intervention be changed or stopped?
- Is there a worsening of the problem, and should the goal and the planned nursing intervention be reviewed?
- Was the goal correctly stated or inappropriate?
- Does the goal require intervention(s) from other members of the healthcare team?

## Summary

- The nursing process forms a framework for practice that provides, a means of setting outcomes, prescribing actions and evaluating results through its five stages: assessment, diagnosis, planning, implementation and evaluation.
- While these stages look sequential, in practice they are interactive and are carried out simultaneously. The nursing process needs to be used with a model of care.

# References

Aggleton, P & Chalmers, H (1986) *Nursing Models and the Nursing Process*. Macmillan Press, London.

Aggleton, P & Chalmers, H (2000) *Nursing Models and Nursing Practice*, 2nd edition. Palgrave, Hampshire.

Aspinall, M J (1976) Nursing diagnosis – the weak link. *Nursing Outlook* 24 (7): 433–7.

Bonney, V & Rothberg, J (1963) *Nursing Diagnosis and Therapy: An Instrument for Evaluation and Measurement*. National League for Nursing, Department of Hospital Nursing, New York.

Crouch, A & Meurier, C (2005) *Vital Notes for Nurses: Health Assessment*. Blackwell Publishing, Oxford.

Doenges, M E & Moorehouse, M F (2003) *Application of the Nursing Process and Nursing Diagnosis*, 4th edition. F A Davis Company, Philadelphia.

George, J B (1990). *Nursing Theories. The Base for Professional Nursing Practice*, 3rd edition. Appleton and Lange, Norwalk, Connectiut.

Hall, L E (1955) Quality of nursing care. *Public Health News*, June. New Jersey State Department of Health, New Jersey.

Henderson, V (1960) *Basic Principles of Nursing Care*. International Council of Nurses, London.

Hodgston, R (2002) Managing care. In: Hodgston, R & Simpson, P M (eds) *Foundations of Nursing Practice: Making the Difference*, 2nd edition. Macmillan, Basingstoke.

Johnson, D E (1959) A philosophy of nursing. *Nursing Outlook* 7: 198–200.

McFarlane, J & Castledine, G (1982) *A Guide to the Practice of Nursing Using the Nursing Process.* C V Mosby, London.

Mundinger, M O & Jauron, G D (1975) Developing a nursing diagnosis. *Nursing Outlook* 23: 94–8.

Orem, D E (1959) *Guides for Developing Curricula for the Education of Practical Nurses.* Government Printing Office, Washington, DC.

Orlando, I J (1961) *The Dynamic Nurse–Patient Relationship: Function, Process and Principles.* G P Putman's Sons, New York. Reprinted 1990, National League for Nursing, New York.

Peplau, H E (1969) Professional closeness: As a special kind of involvement with a patient, client, or family groups. *Nursing Forum* 8: 342–60.

Roper, N, Logan, W & Tierney, A (1980) *The Elements of Nursing*, 1st edition. Churchill Livingstone, Edinburgh.

Roper, N, Logan, W & Tierney, A (2002) *The Elements of Nursing*, 4th edition. Churchill Livingstone, Edinburgh.

Roy, C (1975) *The Roy Adaptation Model.* Prentice-Hall, Englewood Cliffs, New Jersey.

Tierney, A J (1998) Nursing models: extant or extinct? *Journal of Advanced Nursing* 28 (1): 77–85.

Torres, G (1990) The place of concepts and theories within nursing. In: George, J B (ed.) *Nursing Theories: The Base for Professional Nursing Practice*, 3rd edition. Appleton & Lange, Norwalk, Connecticut.

Wiedenbach, E (1963) The helping art of nursing. *American Journal of Nursing* 63: 54–7.

Yura, H & Walsh, M B (1967) *The Nursing Process: Assessing, Planning, Implementing, Evaluating*, 1st edition. Appleton–Century–Crofts, Norwalk, Connecticut.

# Principles of Nursing Practice

# Essence of care and individualised nursing

## Introduction

This chapter will discuss the principles of both 'essence of care' and individualised care. In particular, the concepts of primary nursing and the named nurse will be presented in the context of healthcare delivery.

## Essence of Care

*Essence of Care* is a UK government initiative, which was introduced with the specific remit of helping to improve the quality of patient care. It was developed out of the *Making a Difference* document (Department of Health, 1999) and aimed to introduce clinical practice benchmarking in health care. Essentially, it is a toolkit to support clinical governance; it was originally aimed at eight fundamental aspects of care. It is a patient-focused, good practice guide and is a structured approach to enable clinicians to share and compare good practice. It is also intended to determine methods of measuring continuous quality improvement.

*Essence of Care* was introduced at a time of increasing general dissatisfaction with health care and an acknowledgement by the government that there were unacceptable variations in standards of care across the country (Department of Health, 2000). *Essence of Care* was aimed specifically at ensuring that the fundamental aspects of care meet the needs of patients. Initially eight areas of fundamental aspects of care were identified; these are often referred to as domains of care (Box 5.1). Following further consultation, a further domain, communication, was introduced in 2003, and in 2006, a tenth domain, promoting health, was added.

The initial eight areas were drawn from areas of concern and were identified from complaints by patients, ombudsman reports and from feedback from voluntary organisations, patients, carers and staff. They were very much focused on the fundamentals of care, this was as a result of the general opinion that standards of essential care were slipping.

---

**Box 5.1 Essence of Care domains (Department of Health, 2001).**

(1) Food and nutrition
(2) Privacy and dignity
(3) Continence/bladder/bowel care
(4) Pressure ulcers
(5) Personal and oral hygiene
(6) Safety of patients with mental health needs
(7) Record keeping
(8) Principles of self-care
(9) Communication (added in 2003)
(10) Promoting health (added in 2006)

---

**Activity**

- How important do you think it is that nurses ensure that the most basic aspects of care are right for the patient?
- How do you think the aims of *Essence of Care* can be achieved?
- Where do you find standards for the care you provide?
- Why is it important to develop a structured approach to delivering best practice?

## Benchmarking

In the *Making a Difference* document (Department of Health, 1999, p. 49) clinical practice benchmarking is defined as: 'A process through which best practice is identified and continuous improvement pursued through comparison and sharing'.

*Essence of Care* benchmarks provide a comprehensive set of explicit standards by which the fundamental and essential aspects of care can be measured. The primary concern was the quality of the patient's experience and, to strengthen this, the domains were developed with patient and public involvement at every stage of the consultation. This patient focus is an important aspect of the initiative as it seeks to determine what it is that patients want from health care. *Essence of Care* benchmarking is a process of comparing, sharing and developing practice in order to achieve and sustain best practice (Department of Health, 2001). Changes and improvements focus on the indicators for each domain; these are based on aspects of care that patients, carers and professionals believe are important in achieving best practice. They were intended for use at a local level to ensure improvement in local care delivery. All benchmarking tools are widely available and can be accessed from the Department of Health website (www.dh.gov. uk/Policyandguidance).

The benchmarking cycle is a practical guide, which is easy to use, and extensive guidance is provided. The benchmarking cycle is described below and Table 5.1 outlines each of the phases of the cycle. The tool is designed so that comparison can take place at a number of different levels; from practitioner/ward team level, right through to national services. According to Codling (1995), the real benefits of benchmarking are that it provides a structured approach for comparison and sharing, which can support realistic development.

A key purpose of this approach is to identify good practice, which can then be shared with others. Learning from, and sharing with, the work of others is a very practical and valuable way of improving the quality of patient care, which can be achieved on a local and national level.

### *Benchmarking cycle*

The starting point is to decide on the area of practice that is to be assessed. It is useful to do this in the context of issues and problems. For example, are there any concerns around a particular area of practice? It is also useful to look at the information available regarding the quality of patient care in a particular area.

The stages involved in benchmarking are highlighted in Table 5.1.

**Table 5.1** The benchmarking process (Department of Health, 2001).

| Stage | Description |
| --- | --- |
| Stage 1: Agree best practice | • Consider the patients' or carers' experiences and outcomes, and how current care is delivered<br>• Agree clinical benchmarks to be considered<br>• Establish a comparison group<br>• Consider the overall outcome and the benchmarks of best practice<br>• Using the general indicators and specific indicators agree the evidence that the comparison group consider necessary to be provided in order to achieve the benchmarks of best practice |
| Stage 2: Assess clinical area against best practice | • Obtain baseline information by observing against best practice, using audit and involving patients in the clinical area<br>• Consider the indicators and provide evidence that represents current achievement towards best practice<br>• Consider barriers that prevent achievement of best practice<br>• Compare and share best practice so that good practice is not wasted<br>• Some comparison groups find considering their positions on an E (poor practice) to A (best practice) continuum useful to stimulate discussion |
| Stage 3: Produce and implement action plan aimed at achieving best practice | • Produce an action plan detailing: who the action plan is aimed at, the changes that need to be made, achieving best practice to improve practice, who is responsible for leading the changes, the time scale in which these should occur<br>• Actions should be realistic, achievable and measurable<br>• Carry out the action plan |
| Stage 4: Review achievement towards best practice | • Document activities, any improvement towards best practice problems and or unexpected observations<br>• Analyse data and evaluate actions<br>Did the patients' or carers' experiences or outcomes improve?<br>Did service delivery benefit from changes made?<br>• If there is no improvement, review activities in action plan<br>• Share with comparison group |
| Stage 5: Disseminate improvements and/ or review action plan | • If improvements are identified, disseminate improvements and good practice and implement change widely, or review action plan as appropriate, through comparison group and other organisational systems<br>• Include in organisation's business planning cycle, clinical governance plan and quality report via relevant managers, and clinical governance and quality leads |
| Stage 6/1: Agree best practice | • As stage one |

Broadly the stages of the benchmarking process are

- Stage 1: Agree best practice
- Stage 2: Assess clinical area against best practice
- Stage 3: Produce and implement an action plan aimed at achieving best practice
- Stage 4: Review achievement towards best practice
- Stage 5: Disseminate improvements and/or review action plan
- Stage 6/1: Agree best practice

## Example: Privacy and dignity

*Essence of Care* is all about getting the basics right to improve the patient care experience, but what is a good patient experience? Each *Essence of Care* domain has an agreed patient-focused outcome, for privacy and dignity this outcome is: 'Patients benefit from care that is focused upon respect for the individual'.

There are seven factors with which to benchmark privacy and dignity outlined in the *Essence of Care* toolkit (Department of Health, 2001); they are listed in Table 5.2.

Patients benefit from care that is focused upon the respect of the individual (Woogara, 2004). This respect includes the appropriate use of communication and listening skills, creating the right environment, being responsive to patients' needs and remembering the basics.

---

### Activity: Case study

You are working on an elderly care ward. The ward is very busy, you are tired and you feel you have worked very hard since coming on duty. You are just about to go on your break. The buzzer goes in one of the ward areas. You really want to go on your break, but instead you answer it. The patient is tearful and distressed. He knows you are busy, but he asked someone, he does not know who, to help him use the toilet, but they have not returned. Take a moment to think about how this patient feels.

- How important do you think it is to introduce yourself to patients?
- How long do you think patients should wait for the toilet?
- When carrying out care do you ask for consent?
- What do you do to protect patients' modesty?
- What steps can you take to improve dignity in the care you give every day?
- In what ways do you show respect to patients?

---

More information and examples of good and poor practice in relation to privacy and dignity in care can be found at: http://www.dh.gov.uk/PolicyAndGuidance/HealthAndSocialCareTopics/SocialCare/DignityInCare/fs/en

**Table 5.2** Benchmarks for privacy and dignity.

| Factor | Benchmark of best practice |
| --- | --- |
| (1) Attitudes and behaviours | Patients feel that they matter all of the time |
| (2) Personal world and personal identity | Patients experience care in an environment that actively encompasses individual values, beliefs and personal relationships |
| (3) Personal boundaries and space | Patients' personal space is actively promoted by all staff |
| (4) Communicating with staff and patients | Communication between staff and patients takes place in a manner that respects their individuality |
| (5) Privacy of patient, confidentiality of patient information | Patient information is shared, with their consent, to enable care |
| (6) Privacy, dignity and modesty | Patients' care actively promotes their privacy and dignity, and protects their modesty |
| (7) Availability of an area for complete privacy | Patients and/or carers can access an area that safely provides privacy |

# The organisation of nursing care

Binnie & Titchen (1999) reported three styles of practice that influence the way nursing work is defined and the way it influences the focus of nursing practice. They are:

- traditional nursing
- individualised nursing
- patient-centred nursing (see Chapter 7 for more information).

## Traditional care

The traditional system of nursing care involved nurses carrying out allocated tasks. It was the method by which nurses in the UK trained for many years, and is sometimes referred to as task allocation. Essentially, it was a style of nursing concerned with the dutiful completion of a hierarchy of practical tasks (Binnie & Titchen, 1999). It worked by nursing tasks being allocated to nurses according to their grade. The nurse went around the ward completing this task for each patient, e.g. one nurse would perform all of the blood pressures, one nurse would assist with patient hygiene and another would do the dressings. This regimented method ensured that all the tasks on the ward were done in the shortest time possible.

This traditional approach to care has gradually become outdated, as this style of nursing is not an appropriate method of meeting the contemporary and complex demands of health care. Evidence to support this can be found in the findings of a large study in the 1950s (Menzies,

1970), which concluded that this traditional system of care was dysfunctional for both nurses and patients, most significantly because it failed to support the development of personal relationships between nurses and patients. This inability to provide holistic care led to dissatisfaction for both nurses and patients. Further research in the UK in the 1970s suggested that patients who required care that was not part of the routine tasks would often have that care omitted (Binnie & Titchen, 1999). This style of nursing was impersonal, and nurses often lacked autonomy to make decisions about individual patient's care.

## Individualised care

A growing dissatisfaction with task allocation, together with nursing becoming more academic, led to the development of an individualised approach to nursing care. The move towards individualised care started in the USA in the 1950s and 1960s. This coincided with the development of nursing theory and models of nursing, which began to challenge the medical model of health care. This is outlined in Chapter 3. The advent of the nursing process further supported the move towards individualised nursing care. With individual nursing care plans produced for individual patients, the nursing process and primary nursing are often seen as vehicles for implementing individualised care (Waters & Easton, 1999). Radwin & Alster (2002) reported that individualised nursing became an important feature of nursing care that was designed specifically to meet the needs of the patient, as opposed to the traditional systems, which were service-led care. Radwin & Alster (2002, p. 55) defined individualised care as: 'when the nurse knows the patient as a unique individual and tailors nursing care to a patient's experiences; behaviours; feelings and perceptions'. Similarly, Waters & Easton (1999, p. 83) claimed that individualised nursing care:

> Will recognise the uniqueness of a human being, his/her individuality, personality and human frailty. Individualised care will offer patients many different ways of meeting their needs, allow choice and involve the nurse in listening rather than telling.

Pembrey (1980) suggested that individualised care depends upon individual nurses being allocated personal responsibility for the nursing care of specific patients. Initially, patient allocation was introduced in the UK as a replacement for task allocation (Pembrey, 1975). Although this was an improvement from the task-focused method of care, there were still fundamental problems with this system. Binnie & Titchen (1999) point out that allocation was based only on a particular shift and the next shift might have the nurse being allocated to a different set of patients. This resulted in a lack of continuity of care and prevented the nurse from developing a relationship with the patient. Pollock (1988) identified four parts to individualised care:

- getting to know the patient and carer
- building relationships
- showing you care
- getting patients independent.

It was not until the introduction of the nursing process that individualised nursing in the UK really found its purpose. The nursing process was implemented on a national scale (discussed in detail in Chapter 4) and changed the way nurses organised care. This approach was adopted widely; it was as if it had become legislation. The Royal College of Nursing standards document (1981, p. 9) declared: 'The nursing care of each patient should be individually planned, the plan being based on an assessment of individual needs'.

There is strong evidence to suggest that individualised care is highly valued by nurses (Pollock, 1988), patients and families (Henderson, 1997). There are, generally, three methods of nursing that support the delivery of individualised care. They are:

- primary nursing
- team nursing
- named nursing.

---

**Activity**

In the following case studies both patients have been admitted with an acute stroke. There is national guidance on stroke care. Will the care be the same for each patient?

**Case Study 1:** a 50-year-old male, normally fit and well. Works as a manager for a production company. Very active, plays squash, has two dogs at home. Has a large family who visit regularly. He has been on the ward for 1 week, and has become very depressed, not really communicating with anyone. You know that he is normally very chatty and outspoken.

**Case Study 2:** an 80-year-old female. Lives alone, previous history of falls, not coping at home, not looking after self. No family, but a neighbour visits now and again. She is worried about what will happen to her now and cries a lot.

Think about the care for each patient then answer the following questions:

- How will the care for each patient be the same?
- How might it be different?
- How will you provide individualised care for each patient?

**Patients are different . . . and their care should reflect this!**

## Primary nursing

Primary nursing was developed in the USA in the 1960s and is based on the ideas of Lydia Hall from New York (Hall, 1969). It was developed in response to the frustrations with the current systems of organising care and a growing demand for a more personalised service (Manthey, 1980). Primary nursing came to prominence in the UK in the 1980s (Black, 1992). It is an organisational system in which nurses carry out individual assessments of patients' needs and is based on a relationship between specific nurses and specific patients (Manthey *et al.*, 1970). It encourages professionalism in nursing practice and places 24-hour responsibility and accountability for patient care for the whole patient stay on the primary nurse (Pontin, 1999). Anderson & Choi (1980, p. 29) define primary nursing as:

> *A system organised to maximise continuous and comprehensive delivery of nursing care to patients. Emphasis is on one nurse having professional/organisational autonomy in assuming responsibility and retaining accountability for planning and when possible personally administering total care to designated patients throughout their hospitalisation.*

Primary nursing offers nurses a professional structure in which they have personal responsibility for the nursing care of their own patients (Binnie & Titchen, 1999). Primary nursing is characterised by ten elements, outlined by Watt & O'Leary (1980):

- accountability
- advocacy
- assertiveness
- authority
- autonomy
- collaboration
- communication
- commitment
- continuity
- coordination.

There is some debate in the literature as to whether primary nursing is simply a method to organise the delivery of care, or whether it is also a philosophy of care (Pontin, 1999). For the purpose of this section, it will be discussed as a system of care delivery.

Evidence to support primary nursing suggests that it improves the quality of care, and increases satisfaction of patients and nurses (Rigby *et al.*, 2001). There is evidence to support the claim that it improves the continuity of care, support for staff and improved communication (MacGuire, 1989; Flowers, 1992). There is, however, also some evidence to suggest that it is difficult to measure the benefits of primary nursing, with many studies being inconclusive (Thomas *et al.*, 1996; Rigby *et al.*, 2001). Primary nursing is often considered as an ideal way of delivering care but, in reality, it is difficult to achieve in practice. This is attributed to constraints of staffing levels and skills mixes (Rigby *et al.*, 2001).

## Team nursing

Waters (1985) describes team nursing as a method of allocating a group of nurses to a group of patients. A team leader is responsible for allocating work and for the supervision of the team. Using this system, nurses should still be able to provide individualised nursing; however, there is some debate that this system may support task allocation, with the tasks being distributed within a smaller group of staff. To some extent, this was a more popular alternative to primary nursing in the UK. It was considered a more practical alternative, which still advocated individualised care, but was not as difficult to implement in relation to the perceived number of nurses required to carry out the system of care.

## Named nursing

The concept of named nursing was introduced in *The Patients' Charter* in October 1991. The charter stated that:

> *The charter standard is that you should have a named, qualified nurse, midwife or health visitor who will be responsible for your nursing and midwifery care* (Department of Health, 1991, p. 15).

Named nursing is the advocated approach to delivering individualised care and can exist within both primary nursing and team nursing systems. It is probable that the named nurse concept actually originated from the concept of primary nursing.

The idea of appointing a named nurse to each patient first emerged in a government publication: *A Strategy for Nursing* (Department of Health, 1989). It was perceived as a top-down approach, which was imposed on staff from above and, as a result, attracted criticism as a public relations exercise (Jack, 1995). Despite these initial reservations, the concept of the named nurse appears to be well integrated into care across the UK.

The publication *The Named Nurse, Midwife and Health Visitor: Raising the Standard, Citizens Charter* (Department of Health, 1993) stated that the named nurse should 'ensure that his/her name and responsibilities are known to the patients' and that the named nurse should 'work in partnership' with the patient. Wright (1993) identified the basic principles of named nursing as follows: the named nurse should assess, plan and evaluate care for the named patients. He saw this as an essential element of the named nursing concept and suggested that unless a nurse is involved in this process he or she cannot/should not be the named nurse. A named nurse must be accountable and responsible for coordinating the overall plan of nursing care for the patient.

The named nurse concept stresses the importance of individualised care for patients and places emphasis on the individual relationship with patients (Turner, 1997). Potinkara & Paunonen (1996) investigated factors that help to alleviate anxiety in patients' significant others in a critical care setting and concluded that the patient's named nurse had an important role to play in improving the quality of nursing care. Furthermore, a study by Thomas *et al.* (1996) concluded that patients who could identify a nurse in charge of their care reported more positive experiences of that care. This was irrespective of whether the care was delivered through primary or team nursing.

Continuity of care is of central importance to the named nurse concept and appears to be the key to its success. Melville (1995) acknowledged that patients are empowered when they contribute to their own care planning, but recognises that this is often hindered by traditional attitudes. Procter (1995) argued that the introduction of the named nurse recognises the importance of the continuity of the carer, rather than simply continuity of care. She believed that this is fundamental to the development of therapeutic interpersonal relationships with patients.

### Summary

- *Essence of Care* was introduced by the Department of Health to improve the quality of patient care. It is aimed at the basics of care and provides a detailed toolkit to benchmark good and poor practice.
- The way in which nursing care is organised has changed over time from task allocation to individualised care. Individualised care acknowledges that patients are different and all patients should have an individual assessment of their needs and an individual care plan should be produced.
- Systems of delivering individualised care include primary nursing, team nursing and named nursing.

**A cautionary note: attaching a nurse's name to a group of patients does not constitute individualised care!**

## References

Anderson, M & Choi, T (1980) Primary nursing in an organisational context. *Journal of Nursing Administration* 10: 26–30.

Binnie, A and Titchen, A (1999) *Freedom to Practice: The Development of Patient-Centred Nursing.* Butterworth Heinemann, Oxford.

Black, F (1992) *Primary Nursing: An Introductory Guide*. Kings Fund Centre, London.

Codling, S (1995) *Best Practice Benchmarking: A Management Guide*. Gower, Aldershot.

Department of Health (1989) *A Strategy for Nursing: A Report from the Steering Committee*. Department of Health, Nursing Division, London.

Department of Health (1991) *The Patients Charter*. HMSO, London.

Department of Health (1993) *The Named Nurse, Midwife and Health Visitor: Raising the Standard, Citizens Charter*. HMSO, London.

Department of Health (1999) *Making a difference*. The Stationery Office, London.

Department of Health (2000) *The NHS Plan: A Plan for Investment. A Plan for Reform*. The Stationery Office, London.

Department of Health (2001) *Essence of Care*. The Stationery Office, London.

Flowers, N (1992) Testing Ground. *Nursing Times* 88: 34–5.

Hall, L (1969) The Loeb Center for Nursing and Rehabilitation, Montefiore Hospital and Medical Center, Bronx, New York. *International Journal of Nursing Studies* 6: 81–97.

Henderson, S (1997) Knowing the patient and the Impact on Patient Participation: a Grounded Theory Study. *International Journal of Nursing Practice* 3: 111–18.

Jack, B (1995) Using the named nurse system to improve patient care. *Nursing Times* 91 (44): 34–5.

MacGuire, J M (1989) Primary nursing: a better way to care? *Nursing Times* 85: 243–51.

Manthey, M (1980) *The Practice of Primary Nursing*. Blackwell Scientific Publications, Oxford.

Manthey, M, Ciske, K, Robertson, P & Harris, I (1970) Primary nursing. *Nursing Forum* 9 (1): 65–83.

Melville, E (1995) The implementation of the named nurse concept. *Professional Nurse* 10 (12): 800–801.

Menzies, I E P (1970) *The Functioning of Social Systems as a Defence Against Anxiety*. The Tavistock Institute of Human Relations, London.

Pembrey, S M (1975) From work routines to patient assignment: an experiment in ward organisation. *Nursing Times* 71: 1768–72.

Pembrey, S M (1980) *The Ward Sister – Key to Nursing*. Royal College of Nursing, London.

Pollock, L C (1988) The work of community psychiatric nursing. *Journal of Advanced Nursing* 13: 537–45.

Pontin, D (1999) Primary nursing: a mode of care or a philosophy of nursing. *Journal of Advanced Nursing* 29 (3): 584–91.

Potinkara, H & Paunonen, M (1996) Alleviating anxiety in nursing significant others. *Intensive and Critical Care Nursing* 12 (6): 327–34.

Procter, S (1995) Planning for continuity of carer in nursing. *Journal of Nursing Management* 3 (4): 169–75.

Radwin, L E & Alster, K (2002) Individualised nursing care: an empirically generated definition. *International Council For Nurses, International Review* 49: 54–63.

Rigby, A, Leach, C & Greasley, P (2001) Primary nursing: staff perception of changes in ward atmosphere and role. *Journal of Psychiatric and Mental Health Nursing* 8: 525–32.

Royal College of Nursing (1981) *Towards Standards: a Discussion Document.* RCN, London.

Thomas, L, McColl, E, Priest, J & Bond, S (1996) The impact of primary nursing on patient satisfaction. *Nursing Times* 92 (22): 36–8.

Turner, H (1997) Incorporating the named nurse concept into care. *Professional Nurse* 12 (8): 582–4.

Waters, K (1985) Team nursing. *Nursing Practice* 1: 7–15.

Waters, K R & Easton, N (1999) Individualised care: is it possible to plan and carry out? *Journal of Advanced Nursing* 29 (1): 79–87.

Watt, V & O'Leary, J (1980) Ten components of primary nursing. *Nursing Dimensions* 7 (4): 90–95.

Woogara, J (2004) Patients' right to privacy and dignity in the NHS. *Nursing Standard* 19 (18): 33–7.

Wright, S (1993) The named nurse, midwife and health visitor – principles and practices. In: *The Named Nurse, Midwife and Health Visitor: Raising the Standard, Citizens Charter.* HMSO, London.

# Principles of communication 6

## Learning objectives

- Understand the principles of communication.
- Understand the increasing role of participation by patients and their carers in health care.
- Identify effective ways of giving and collecting information.
- Understand the principles and practical issues about consent.
- Identify ways in which the nurse can act as patient advocate and why this is important.
- Understand the principles of ethics and how these affect care delivery.

## Introduction

This chapter will discuss the principles of communication in providing nursing care, which includes patient participation, information giving and sharing, securing consent, patient advocacy and ethics.

All individuals will have been involved in situations where effective and ineffective methods of communication have been used. These experiences highlight the importance of effective communication and how much it affects us, not only in terms of our satisfaction with the product that we might have purchased, but also our overall experience of that situation. It is easy, then, to see how poor communication can affect both the care that patients receive and the way that they view that care. Communication is central to the delivery of effective health care. Effective communication can help build productive relationships between healthcare professionals and patients and their carers. Ineffective communication can result in ineffective care and, not surprisingly, dissatisfied patients. A number of principles underpin effective communication and these will be discussed in this chapter. It is also important to consider the increasing role that patients play in health care and the implications that this has for communication.

## Patient participation

At the time of writing this book, the agenda for healthcare reform is firmly focused on the modernisation of the National Health Service. The NHS plan for England (Department of Health, 2000) proposes important changes in the roles of patients in the health service. The key proposals that address the role of patients within the NHS and patient empowerment are included in Chapter 10 of *The NHS Plan* (Department of Health, 2000) and include: information to empower patients, strengthening patient choice, a new patient advocacy service, rights of redress and patients' views, scrutiny of the NHS, and patient representation throughout the NHS. *The NHS Improvement Plan*, published in June 2004 by the Department of Health, set out the way in which the NHS needs to change in order to become truly patient led. The aim of the current reform is that health care will provide a coordinated, comprehensive and effective system of care that reflects patients' needs.

Evidence indicates that patients want to be treated as individuals, want clear explanations about what is wrong with them, want to know what to expect, and want to be involved in decisions about their care (British Medical Association, 2000). This has implications for the delivery of care and all that this involves, which includes communication.

---

**Activity**

Think about your clinical practice and what the patients that you work with want in relation to their health care.

- From your experiences, what do you believe are the most important issues for patients as consumers?
- Do these issues vary between patients?
- If so, how?
- Is it easy to adapt care to individual needs?

---

Patients are now more involved in the management of health care than has been the case previously. They provide input at an individual level, through discussions about their own care, at organisational levels through membership on patient advisory groups and at a national level by influencing the content of clinical guidelines, such as those compiled by the National Institute for Health and Clinical Excellence (NICE). In addition, there are a number of organisations that promote and support their participation in health care.

One example of this is patient participation groups, who work with general practices to provide practical support, to help patients to take more responsibility for their own health and to provide strategic input and advice. They are based on cooperation between the practice staff and patients and aim to improve communication. These groups are not new, with the first formed in 1972 and the National Association for Patient Participation (NAPP) registered in 1978 as their umbrella organisation. NAPP promotes the concept of self-help and aims to see a patient participation group in every GP practice. It maintains a volunteer network of officers who train practices in setting up local patient participation groups in their locality. Further information can be gained from their website: www.napp.org.uk/

## Communication

It is important to remember that there are, principally, two reasons for communicating: to collect information and to provide information. Nurses are involved in both of these in their daily work.

### *What is communication?*

Communication can be defined as:

> *a two-way process in which information is transmitted and received. It also involves feedback between the recipient and the transmitter of information* (Crouch & Meurier, 2005, p. 129).

The main elements involved in the process of communication are illustrated in Figure 6.1.

---

**Activity**

Think about what communication means to you, and particularly about what effective communication means.

• Define what effective communication means to you.

Think about the way you and your colleagues communicate: (1) with each other; (2) with patients:

• How do you know if this is effective?
• What could you do to ensure that it is?

---

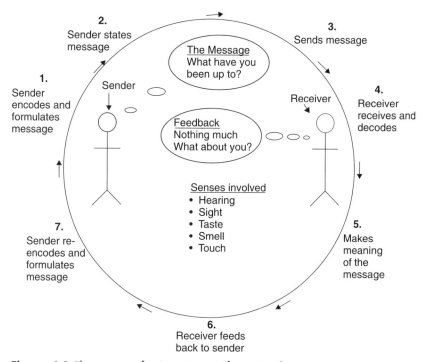

**Figure 6.1** The process of communication (from Crouch & Meurier, 2005, p. 129). Reprinted with permission of Anna Amugi-Crouch.

## Collecting information

Nurses and other healthcare professionals can make use of a range of different communication styles to gain information about patients. This information will include details of a patient's presenting condition, medical history, physiological parameters, physical signs and symptoms, all of which can be ascertained by targeted (head to toe) assessment, observation and directed questions. As well as information about a patient's physical health, it is often necessary to find out about a patient's mental well-being. To gain this information it will be necessary to use structured questions about recent behaviour, to observe the patient and to ask him or her to describe his/her perceptions about this.

Obtaining the views of patients is important in order to gain information about their views of their care, so that they can be involved in, and influence the management of their current and future care. Patient participation, which will be discussed in more detail later in this chapter, is becoming increasingly important in the delivery of health care. There are a number of ways in which the views of patients can be collected. These methods include: one-to-one discussions with the patient, observing and listening to patients, patient satisfaction surveys, patient diaries, user groups, patient panel, seeking feedback from patient advocates or carers, and providing a feedback box on the ward. The most effective method will depend on the situation, with one-to-one discussions more suited to collecting information about an individual and group discussions for views about broader healthcare issues. It is important to remember that, regardless of the method used to collect information, and how well this is done, there is little value in this exercise unless there is accurate documentation of what is collected.

## Confidentiality

Maintaining the confidentiality of patient information is now a well-established practice in health care. The *Caldicott Report* (Department of Health, 1997) was a review commissioned by the Chief Medical Officer at that time to make recommendations to improve the way the NHS handles and protects patient information. It resulted in the introduction of a process of continuous improvement in confidentiality within the NHS, including the organisations that now comprise the Health Protection Agency (HPA). The principles in the *Caldicott Report* are presented in Box 6.1.

Patients have the right to expect that identifiable information about them will not be shared outside the healthcare team responsible for their care unless they have given explicit consent. Therefore, the information that is collected about a patient should be treated as confidential and should not be used for any purpose other than for informing the plan of care needed by that patient. While confidentiality normally refers to the non-sharing of any information, there are situations in health care in which non-identifiable information about the patient can be used without a patient's consent. These include situations when patients are diagnosed with certain diseases, and the HPA gathers

---

**Box 6.1 The principles in the Caldicott Report (Department of Health, 1997).**

(1) Justify the purpose(s) for using patient data.
(2) Don't use patient-identifiable information unless it is absolutely necessary.
(3) Use the minimum necessary patient-identifiable information.
(4) Access to patient-identifiable information should be on a strict need-to-know basis.
(5) Everyone should be aware of their responsibilities to maintain confidentiality.
(6) Understand and comply with the law, in particular the Data Protection Act.

information that is used to improve medical care and to protect the health of others (see http://www.hpa.org.uk/for further information about the role of the HPA).

## *Providing information*

Before patients (and their carers) can make decisions about their care, they need information about their condition and about possible treatments and investigations involved. This should include information about: the risks and benefits of these treatments as well as the risks and benefits of deciding not to have them, and whether other procedures will be necessary as part of these treatments or investigations. It is important that the information given to patients is comprehensible, consistent and of good quality. This highlights the importance of effective communication and documentation by and between healthcare professionals in the provision of information to patients.

The provision of information should not stop when a patient makes a decision about his or her care. Rather, once they have made one or a number of decisions about their care – whether or not to have a particular treatment, for example – patients need information about what this will involve. This includes the practical details of when and where care will be provided, how long they are likely to be in hospital, and how they are likely to feel during and after this, as well as details of what is expected from the particular treatment or investigation and what they should expect to happen as a result.

When providing information, it is important to remember that the amount of information that patients and their carers want will vary considerably. Given the increasing role of patients in their care, it is right to assume that the patient will want to know about the risks and benefits of treatments and investigations. With this in mind, however, nurses will have to make judgements about the nature and amount of information required by the patient in each situation. Some patients will want as much detail as possible, some will want to know some detail but only to a specified level, some will want to know the bare minimum, and some will ask you as a nurse, or another health professional, to make a decision or decisions for them. The level of information that is provided to the patient is something that needs to be negotiated and agreed between the health professional and the patient. In situations where the patient indicates that he or she does not wish to be given information, this should be documented (Department of Health, 2002). It is important to remember that withholding information is not appropriate. It is also important to remember that other members of the multi-professional team should be consulted when providing information to patients, particularly when this is of a sensitive nature.

As well as the information that is provided by members of the healthcare team, there are a number of other ways in which patients can access information about their condition and its treatment. These include information provided by healthcare organisations, including the NHS, and other disease-specific organisations, such as the British Heart Foundation. If there is a need to produce information for patients, there are a number of resources available that can be used to produce written information for patients, including a toolkit for producing patient information (available online at http://www.nhsidentity.nhs.uk/patientinformationtoolkit/patientinfotoolkit.pdf)

Where information is not provided, and even if it is, some patients will search for more information about their condition and its treatment. Sources will include peer-reviewed information, such as that on recognised websites, such as the Department of Health and patient information websites providing information about health, disease, illness and related medical information (such as: http://www.patient.co.uk/). There is also the potential that patients will obtain information from other sources such as friends, neighbours, websites that produce information that is not peer-reviewed. It is important that any perceptions about their condition and its treatment are discussed and any misconceptions resolved.

When providing information to help patients make choices about their health care, it is important to consider that the choices they make are likely to be affected by a number of factors, which include their willingness and capability to take responsibility for decisions about their health. This is particularly important in a system of health care that is putting increasing emphasis on the contribution of patients to their own health. Each individual's ability to participate in their health care can be determined by the nature of healthcare provision (Pooley *et al.*, 2003), their socio-economic status (SES) (Woodward *et al.*, 2003), their health literacy (Schillinger *et al.*, 2002), their gender (Schoenberg *et al.*, 2003) and their health status (Riegel & Carlson, 2002). In addition, many patients believe in the power of others to control and manage their health. This is illustrated by the old adage 'doctor knows best'. It is also important to remember that there are some who do not wish to accept responsibility for decisions regarding their health and that, regardless of the information they receive, will choose not to do so.

---

**Activity**

Think about how you provide information.

- How do you know if a patient has correctly understood what you have said?
- What methods could you use to make sure this is the case?

# Securing consent

While the provision of information ensures that patients can make informed choices about their health care, it also enables them to give informed consent to any treatment(s) or investigation(s).

## *What is consent?*

Before a patient undergoes any examination, treatment or any aspect of care, he or she must give consent or permission. This includes simple procedures, such as taking a patient's blood pressure or heart rate, more invasive procedures, such as blood taking and skin biopsies, and more invasive tests and treatments, such as complex medical treatments and surgery. Consent can be obtained in a number of ways and these are determined by the severity of the proposed treatment or care. It is important to remember that the way in which consent is obtained is less important than ensuring that consent is informed. For example, a patient might indicate his or her consent to having a blood pressure check by rolling up a sleeve and lifting his/her arm. For more serious treatments involving risks and benefits, he or she might indicate consent by signing a consent form. What is important in all situations (Department of Health, 2002) is that the patient:

- is able to give his or her consent
- is given enough information to enable him or her to make an informed decision
- must be acting under his or her own free will, without strong influence of another person.

The Nursing and Midwifery Council's *Code of Professional Conduct* (2002) addresses the issue of consent. It recognises the importance of informed consent and highlights the importance of protecting patient autonomy and also of ensuring that accurate information is provided about the treatment, investigation or other care patients might need. The implementation of these without adequate consent is not considered lawful. It is an established part of law that treatment cannot be given unless the patient concerned has consented. If health-care professionals proceed without such consent, they are liable to be sued by the patient (even if no harm was done) or to criminal prosecution.

---

**Activity**

Think about what consent means to you.

- Can you define consent, or state what it means to give consent?
- If you have ever had to provide consent yourself, what was the experience like?
- What do you think it is like for patients?

Think about the way you gain consent from patients:

- Do you think this is always effective and that patients are truly informed?
- What could be improved?

---

## *How to obtain consent*

In order to ensure that the consent process becomes focused on the rights of patients and their carers, *The NHS Plan* (Department of Health, 2000) identifies a need for changes to the way in which patients are asked to give their consent to treatment, care or research. The aim of this is to ensure that the rights of each patient are recognised and that the process of seeking consent must enable patients to make healthcare choices that are right for them. It is important to remember that different patients will make different choices at different times, even if they are in apparently similar situations. Healthcare professionals must remain aware of their need to respect individual decisions. It is imperative that they remain objective, and do not make value judgements regarding patients' choices about health care.

In considering individual responses to health care, it might be helpful to reflect on your own beliefs about health care and on the literature surrounding health beliefs, which holds that every patient has unique circumstances, beliefs and ways of responding. Culture, ethnicity and tradition influence beliefs about health and illness. They shape the decisions made by individuals to protect, maintain or promote health and can also cause them to neglect or jeopardise their health. One example that might provide an opportunity to reflect on personal health beliefs is the overwhelming evidence against suntans, especially in relation to sunbathing and the use of sun beds, and that, despite this, suntans continue to represent affluence and are considered a status symbol in the UK.

**Activity**

Think about your own beliefs and behaviour about sunbathing:

*   If you are on a summer holiday and in the sun, do you sunbathe and hope to return with a suntan?
*   Do you think it is important to have tanned skin?
*   If so, why?
*   Do you wear sunscreen?

*   Does the same apply to children?
*   How do your answers compare?

In relation to the ability of an individual to provide consent, English law assumes that if you're an adult you are able to make your own decisions, unless it is proved otherwise. As long as you understand and evaluate the information you need to make the decision, you should be able to do so. There are, however, situations where this will not be the case and other ways of gaining consent are required. The New Model documentation, developed as part of the Department of Health's *Good Practice in Consent* initiative (Department of Health, 2001), addresses this by the publication of the following consent forms:

*Consent form 1*: for patients able to consent for themselves.
*Consent form 2*: for those with parental responsibility, consenting on behalf of a child or young person.
*Consent form 3*: both for patients able to consent for themselves and for those with parental responsibility consenting on behalf of a child/young person, where the procedure does not involve any impairment of consciousness.
*Consent form 4*: for use where the patient is an adult unable to consent to investigation or treatment.

The Department of Health has also published a range of guidance documents on consent, which are freely available from www.doh.gov.uk/consent and include:

*   *Reference guide to consent for examination or treatment*, March 2001
*   *12 key points on consent: the law in England*, March 2001
*   *Consent – what you have a right to expect*, July 2001 (leaflet for patients, with versions for adults, children/young people, people with learning disabilities, parents and relatives/carers)
*   *Seeking consent: working with children*, November 2001
*   *Seeking consent: working with older people*, November 2001
*   *Seeking consent: working with people with learning disabilities*, November 2001

# Ethics

Ethics has been defined as 'the moral principles governing or influencing conduct' (*Oxford English Dictionary*, 2001, p. 490). According to Beauchamp & Childress (1994) ethics is a generic term for various ways of examining moral life. This, in turn, refers to conventions about the rights and wrongs of human conduct; in other words morality. Gillon (1986) proposes four ethical principles, which have been adopted in health care:

(1)  Autonomy; independence to determine one's own direction with the only condition being the need to respect others' individual liberties. This is referred to by Gillon (1986) as the capacity to think and to decide and act on the basis of such thought, and decide freely and independently without hindrance. In health care, the patient's capacity to think and to make deliberate decisions is often hindered. Patients are often in pain, frightened and hypoxic, and therefore have a reduced capacity to decide for themselves. Autonomy requires practitioners to obtain consent for treatment and care and to treat patient information as confidential.

(2)  Beneficence; the righteous philosophy of doing good.

(3)  Non-maleficence, where duty requires no harm to be done.

Principles (2) and (3) are often considered together as, whenever we try to help others, we inevitably risk harming them. Practitioners must ensure that the ultimate aim of care or treatment is that of benefit over harm. The traditional Hippocratic moral obligation of medicine reflects this; that is, beneficence with non-maleficence.

(4)  Justice – often regarded as synonymous with fairness. Gillon (1986) subdivides the obligations of justice into three categories:
   (a)  distributive justice: the fair distribution of scarce resources
   (b)  rights-based justice: respect for people's rights
   (c)  legal justice: respect for morally acceptable laws.

Gillon (1986) asserts that all four principles should be underpinned by respect and the value of human life. While these principles cannot guide clinical judgements or decisions in isolation, they comprise an extremely useful tool.

# Patient advocacy

Ethics, which focuses on issues of duty and responsibility, underpins healthcare delivery. Ethics extends beyond knowledge of ethical codes and conduct to include the ability to discriminate and make moral judgements in complex situations. This involves acting as an advocate for others. It is important to remember that while illness, disease, disability and infirmity may interfere with patients' ability to make choices, they do not alter their right to do so, nor their right to make choices that are right for them. Patient advocacy, a responsibility often assumed by the nurse, provides a means of transferring authority back to the patient. Advocacy is based on the development of the nurse–patient relationship and a resultant partnership that focuses on agreed healthcare goals. This enables the nurse to understand the patient's values, priorities and expectations. Brown's (1985) view of patient advocacy, which stresses the importance of disclosing both benefits and possible adverse effects of all treatments, as well as the alternative therapies available, still applies today. With such knowledge, patient decisions are both informed and autonomous.

## Summary

- Effective communication is fundamental to effective health care.
- The importance of good communication has been highlighted by the increasing role of patients in health care.
- Without effective communication, patients are not adequately informed about their care, informed consent is not possible and their wishes are not recognised.
- Ineffective communication between healthcare professionals has implications for care delivery and can have a negative impact on patient care.

# References

Beauchamp, T L & Childress, J F (1994) *Principles of Biomedical Ethics.* Oxford University Press, New York, USA.

British Medical Association (2000) What sort of healthcare does the public expect, want or need? *Healthcare Funding Review Research Report Summary.* Available at www.bma.org.uk/ap.nsf/Content/ Healthcare+ funding+review+research+report+1.

Brown, M (1985) Matter of commitment. *Nursing Times* 81 (18): 26–7.

Crouch, A & Meurier, C (2005) *Vital Notes for Nurses: Health Assessment.* Blackwell Publishing, Oxford.

Department of Health (1997) *The Caldicott Committee Report on the Review of Patient-Identifiable Information.* Available at http://www.dh.gov.uk/asset-Root/04/06/84/04/04068404.pdf.

Department of Health (2000) *The NHS Plan. A Plan for investment, A plan for reform.* Secretary of State for Health. The Stationery Office, London.

Department of Health (2001) *Good Practice in Consent: Achieving the NHS Plan Commitment to Patient-Centred Consent Practice*. The Stationery Office, London.

Department of Health (2002) *Good Practice in Consent Implementation Guide*. Available at http://www.dh.gov.uk/assetRoot/04/01/90/61/04019061.pdf.

Department of Health (2004) *The NHS Improvement Plan: Putting People at the Heart of Public Services*. Available at http://www.dh.gov.uk/asset-Root/04/08/45/22/04084522.pdf.

Gillon, R (1986) *Philosophical Medical Ethics*. Chichester, Wiley.

Nursing and Midwifery Council (2002) *Code of Professional Conduct*. NMC, London.

*Oxford English Dictionary* (2001) Oxford University Press, Oxford.

Pooley, C G, Briggs, J, Gatrell, T, Mansfield, T, Cummings D & Deft, J (2003) Contacting your GP when the surgery is closed: issues of location and access. *Health and Place* 9: 23–32.

Riegel, B & Carlson, B (2002) Facilitators and barriers to heart failure self-care. *Patient Education and Counselling* 46: 287–95.

Schillinger, D, Grumbach, K, Piette, J, Wang, F & Osmond D (2002) Association of health literacy with diabetes outcomes. *Journal of the American Medical Association* 288 (4): 475–82.

Schoenberg, N E, Peters, J C & Drew E M (2003) Unravelling the mysteries of timing: women's perceptions about time for treatment for cardiac symptoms. *Social Science and Medicine* 56: 271–84.

Woodward, M, Oliphant, J, Lowe, G & Tunstall-Pedoe, H (2003) Contribution of contemporaneous risk factors to social inequality in coronary heart disease and all causes mortality. *Preventive Medicine* 36: 561–8.

# 7

# Developing
# therapeutic relationships

## Learning objectives

- Understand the principles of therapeutic relationships.
- Recognise the important of therapeutic nursing in everyday nursing practice.
- Identify ways in which nurses can work in partnerships with patients.
- Understand the benefits of patient-centred nursing.
- Identify a number of defence mechanisms that patients might exhibit.

## Introduction

This chapter will discuss the principles of developing therapeutic relationships with patients and how partnerships with patients are important. The way that therapeutic relationships relate to nursing models and the evidence for, and challenges of, the concept of patient-centred nursing will also be discussed. Finally, aspects of counselling, including recognising defence mechanisms in patients, will be presented.

The demands of modern health care require nurses to perform roles that were traditionally carried out in the medical domain. This has led to a recent domination of clinical skills development in nursing practice. Understandably, this is both an exciting and challenging time for nurses; however, this should not be viewed merely as a move towards developing nurses into 'mini' doctors. Nursing, as a profession, has many unique skills, which have developed over many years; these are reflected in nursing theory and embedded in nursing practice. It is important to remember that nursing is concerned with relationships, with both patients and colleagues (Freshwater, 2003). It is paramount that these skills continue to be promoted and supported. One of the most important of these is the development of therapeutic relationships with patients.

# Therapeutic relationships

As discussed in Chapter 5, it is possible for patient care to be delivered irrespective of patients' individual needs. For example, all patients with the same condition on a particular ward may receive exactly the same care. This care may meet the basic needs of the patient's condition, but it is not patient-centred, it is what can be termed institutionalised nursing. It is only through developing therapeutic relationships with patients that care can be truly patient centred. Nurses need to know what patients' individual needs are in order to best work with them to achieve these goals.

## *Therapeutic relationships and nursing models*

Therapeutic relationships are concerned with the humanistic aspects of nursing care. They represent individualised care based on a caring relationship. This approach to caring is a common feature of nursing theory, and is central to nursing practice. Some nurse theorists have referred directly to therapeutic relationships in their work. Orem (1995, p. 54) refers to the word therapeutic as being: 'supportive of life processes, remedial or curative when related to malfunction due to disease processes, and contributing to personal development and maturing'.

According to Henderson (1980), nursing practice encompasses the ability of the nurse to develop and use a deep understanding and empathy of an individual's world to increase the efficacy, and ensure the quality, of care. She goes on to assert that this knowledge may be used to develop a 'best' approach to holistic care by making interventions responsive to the needs and circumstances of individual patients.

Of the nursing theorists, Peplau refers most explicitly to defining therapeutic relationships in theoretical terms. She describes four phases of the nurse–patient relationship (Table 7.1). Peplau (1952) emphasises the therapeutic value of the nurse and the patient getting to know each other as people and respecting each other, to work in partnership in the resolution of actual or potential problems.

**Table 7.1** Phases of therapeutic relationships (adapted from Peplau, 1988).

| Phase | Description |
|---|---|
| Orientation | Nurse and client meet as strangers, orientate to each other and establish rapport while working together to clarify and define the existing problem(s). |
| Identification | Client and nurse clarify each other's perceptions and expectations |
| Exploration | Nurse encourages client to take an active responsible role in his or her own therapy |
| Resolution | Termination of the therapeutic relationship, nurse and client become more independent of each other. Original needs are met |

**Activity**

- What do you understand by the term therapeutic relationship?
- How do you think this can be achieved in nursing?
- How could therapeutic relationships assist patients?
- How could therapeutic relationships assist nurses?

## Patients as partners

Muetzel (1988) identified the three elements of partnership, intimacy and reciprocity as being the key concepts of therapeutic relationships in nursing. Of these, partnership has the strongest representation in current healthcare practices. The nursing profession has long embraced the concept of working in partnership with patients, especially in relation to care planning, making choices and becoming involved in their care (Royal College of Nursing, 1987).

The drive by the Department of Health, evident in *The NHS Plan* (Department of Health, 2000) and subsequent white papers, has been to advocate the concept of patients as being partners in their own care and in the provision of care in general. *The NHS Plan* identified short-comings in the service and stated that the NHS would deliver an inte-grated system of care using a person-centred approach, and stated that this would enable better care for the individual. It set objectives to enhance access to services and reduce waiting times, while providing a high quality of care, offering increased choice to patients, raising emphasis on prevention, improved relationships and more and better information at the time patients need it, within a better environment.

At the time of writing this book, the most recent initiatives of working in partnerships with patients are those around patient choice, with particular emphasis on giving patients more freedom in relation to how, when and where they receive their care. Most recently, the NHS has introduced 'choose and book', this is a new service that allows the patient to choose the hospital or clinic they wish to go to and book an appointment with a specialist. Patients are able to choose from at least four hospitals or clinics and they are also able to choose the date and time of their appointment. This is far removed from the traditional system whereby patients were expected to fit in with rigid NHS systems, where patients were given an appointment with little negotiation on when, where and by whom this would be provided (see Chapter 12 for more information on patient choice and 'choose and book').

Many independent patient and care organisations, for example the Patient Association, Action on Epilepsy, the MS Society and the Stroke Association, have long been advocates of the concept of patients being partners in their care. They are a driving force in not only influencing government healthcare policy but also in encouraging individual patients and carers to develop true partnerships in their care, rather than being merely recipients of it.

The concept of patients as partners is also reflected in evidence for best practice throughout a whole range of published research, guidance documents and protocols and procedures. This is particularly reflected in National Institute for Health and Clinical Excellence (NICE) guidance. An example of this is in recent NICE guidance published for epilepsy (NICE, 2004, p. 6), which states that, in terms of management:

> *Healthcare professionals should adopt a consulting style that enables the individual with epilepsy, and their family and/or carers as appropriate, to participate as partners in all decisions about their healthcare, and take fully into account their race, culture and any specific needs.*

## Therapeutic nursing

Central to therapeutic nursing is the concept that the patient is not merely a recipient of care, but an active participant in the process. Engaging the patient in a relationship and in the process of care is crucial to the therapeutic nature of nursing practice. The importance of therapeutic nursing has been widely recognised and a number of models of therapeutic nursing practice have emerged. Ersser (1997) identified the therapeutic nature of nursing as including the following activities:

- interacting and forming a relationship with the patient
- helping with bodily caring
- helping the patient to learn
- influencing the context of care
- being caring.

Sherwood (1997) identified four patterns of therapeutic nursing practice:

(1) Healing interaction, which is concerned with providing a setting beneficial to healing, where nurses demonstrate support and protection.
(2) Nurses' knowledge, involving the use of knowledge of human behaviour to develop skills and communicate positive personal attributes.
(3) Intentional response, this describes the performance by the nurse of caring activities through the organisation and planning of clinical skills.
(4) Therapeutic outcome, this describes the aims of therapeutic nursing practice in terms of patients' relationships with nursing staff and the patient's sense of well-being.

Not surprisingly, continuity of care is central to the development of therapeutic relationships between nurses and patients. When care is organised in a way that does not support continuity of care, it is less likely that these caring relationships are formed. As Binnie & Titchen (1999) explain, when a nurse will not be caring for the same patients the following day, then he/she can never be sure that they can follow up care; it is, therefore, less likely that the nurse will build a therapeutic relationship with the patient. The development of such relationships with patients cannot rely solely on the nurse as an individual. To succeed in delivering therapeutic nursing it is important that the way care is organised supports the development of such relationships. Individualised nursing was discussed in Chapter 5. This system of care is one way in which therapeutic nursing is fostered.

---

**Activity**

- What do you think the barriers are to developing therapeutic relationships with patients?
- What can nurses do to balance the demands of health care organisation with the needs of the individual?

---

## Patient-centred nursing

Binnie & Titchen (1999) argue that although the intention of individualised nursing is to place the needs of the patient at the centre, the way in which work is organised can sometimes prevent the development of relationships and is therefore not truly patient centred. The concept of patient centred nursing (which is sometimes referred to as person-centred nursing) is becoming popular in terms of providing holistic health care for patients.

Patient-centred nursing is about humanising nursing practice and emphasising the interpersonal relationships between nurses and patients. Binnie & Titchen (1999) define patient-centred nursing as a style of practice that demonstrates respect for the patient as a person. Pontin (1999) describes being patient centred as emphasising the comforting and caring aspects of the nursing role. The patient is at the centre of all activity, patients are actively involved in planning their care, and patient records reflect this notion, being patient focused as opposed to professionally led. Patient-centred nursing care supports the development of therapeutic relationships between nurses and patients, with patients viewed as playing a vital and active part in their recovery, in which they are encouraged to take control of and responsibility for their health.

McCormack (2001) describes person-centredness as being concerned with the authenticity of the individual. He argues that it is the values and beliefs of individuals that makes them unique, and person-centred nursing acknowledges this. To be person centred, nurses must acknowledge individuals' beliefs, values, wants, needs and desires. They must also be able develop relationships with patients by using approaches that enable flexibility, mutuality, respect and care (McCormack, 2001).

Person centredness is not exclusively a nursing domain, but increasingly central to all healthcare provision. The concept has been studied in relation to dental care (Nestel & Betson, 1999) and GP practice (Mead & Bower, 2000). In fact, its origins can be traced back much further than this, for example this quote from Mahatma Gandhi who is responsible for the following Bombay hospital motto:

*A patient is the most important person in our Hospital. He is not an interruption to our work, he is the purpose of it. He is not an outsider in our Hospital, he is a part of it. We are not doing a favour by serving him, he is doing us a favour by giving us an opportunity to do so.*

## Support

There are many documented benefits of this approach to nursing care, for both patients and nurses; however, much of this is anecdotal evidence. A more holistic approach to care was reported by Binnie & Titchen (1999) in an action research study, which used practice development to implement patient-centred nursing in an acute medical unit. Other reported benefits include increased patient satisfaction with the level of care, reduction in anxiety levels among nurses and increased job satisfaction. Research that has tested the effectiveness of patient-centred nursing has not been able to attribute person-centred nursing directly to improvements in care (Thomas et al., 1996).

## Challenges

The relationship between the nurse and the patient in therapeutic nursing is one of negotiation (unless adverse circumstance mean otherwise). The nurse's role is to empower patients, encouraging them to take responsibility for regaining their health, and utilising the nurse as a resource to achieve this (McMahon & Pearson, 1998). However, as a consequence of the way that health care is organised, patients are often defined by their health problems. Various health professionals each work with a particular problem, for example, a physiotherapist may work with the patient to help him/her to learn to walk again, a dietician may work with the patient to help him/her lose weight, and a doctor may work with the patient to treat his/her high blood pressure. Of all the professions, nurses are best placed to develop therapeutic relationships with patients, to be able to work with them in a holistic way and to guide them through the challenges and choices they face, with regard not only to their health but also to how health care is organised.

---

**Activity**

Think for a moment of all the health professionals involved in patient care.

- How many have 'therapist' in their title?
- How does their role differ from the role of the nurse?
- What distinct contribution do you think you can make as a nurse to patient care?
- Make a list of skills you think nurses need, to be able to develop therapeutic relationships with patients.

---

Some consider nursing as a therapy (McMahon & Pearson, 1998). The skills and behaviour of nurses in developing relationships certainly support the concept of nursing as a therapy. There are many skills required by nurses to enable them to engage in therapeutic relationships with patients. These include sharing, comforting, teaching, informing and communicating (Wright, 1998). Likewise, Burton (2000) suggests that some nursing interventions lead to a more meaningful degree of interaction between the patient and nurse; these include helping, comforting, teaching and working with the patient and family.

The emphasis for patient-centred nursing is that not only are the skills important, but also the way in which the skills are carried out. It is important to work with the patient, alongside him/her, allowing the patient to make his/her own decisions, or to act as the patient's advocate if the patient is unable to make decisions for him/herself. The nurse must have the ability to stand back and guide the patient. This may sound simple, but sometimes it is difficult for nurses to do this. Because of the continued influences of traditional nurse training, and the way nursing work is organised, nurses often want to 'come up with the solution', 'to make the patient better', 'to fix it'. However, in therapeutic nursing the nurse must remember that the patient must direct the outcome, guided by the nurse.

To some extent therapeutic nursing is at odds with the current drive towards greater technology, more clinical skills focused nursing. Wright (1998) argues that some of the most important therapeutic nursing activities are undervalued and seen as menial. He asserts that these 'high-touch' skills in nursing, as opposed to 'high-tech' skills, are important to the delivery of patient-centred care.

## Counselling

Nurses need to develop self-awareness and interpersonal and emotional skills (Freshwater, 2003). There is some debate about the definition of counselling and this has led to debate about whether nurses actually counsel. The general agreement seems to be that although nurses are not counsellors, they do use counselling skills. Counselling, as defined by the British Association for Counselling and Psychotherapy, is:

> *An interaction in which one person offers another person time; attention and respect, with the intention of helping that person explore, discover and clarify ways of living more successfully and towards greater well being* (Palmer *et al.*, 1996, p. 22).

Furthermore, Soohbany (1999) discusses the similarities between nursing and counselling, describing both as an interpersonal process in assisting the individual to cope with life events. In particular, it is the caring element of the role in which counselling and nursing overlap, both being essentially therapeutic in nature.

In part, the work of psychologists, such as Carl Rogers, have influenced the development of patient-centred nursing. Rogers (1967) advocated a style of therapeutics in which the patient is valued as a person, and the key characteristics of the relationship are of the therapist being open and genuine, helping the patient towards psychological growth and well-being. This is more commonly known as 'unconditional positive regard'. The important aspect of this approach for nursing is that the style of counselling fits very well with the development of a therapeutic relationship with the patient. The nurse is not deemed the expert, offering solutions, but rather the nurse assists the individual to find his/her own solutions, and in this non-directive approach, the patient becomes an active partner in his/her care (Binnie & Titchen, 1999).

## Defence mechanisms

Person-centred care involves a level of openness and honesty in relationships with patients (Barber, 1999). It is important for nurses to be aware of their own feelings and reactions, to let down their own defences (Rogers, 1983). Resolving and working through defence mechanisms is an important aspect of the therapeutic relationship. Barber (1999) suggests that nurses should be familiar with more common defence behaviours in order to be able to work with the patient in addressing them (Table 7.2).

Nurses have a duty to adopt therapeutic nursing as a focus of their activity in order to provide best care for the patient (McMahon & Pearson, 1998). However, the environment in which nurses work must be supportive of this concept if is to be effective.

**Table 7.2** Common defence behaviours (adapted from Barber, 1999, p. 177).

| Behaviour | Description |
| --- | --- |
| Repression | The exclusion from awareness of a painful or stress-inducing thought, feeling, memory or impulse |
| Denial | Discarding or transforming an emotive event in such a way that it appears to be unrecognisable |
| Rationalisation | Reasoning is employed to deflect from the emotional significance of an event |
| Identification | Be like or assume the personality characteristics of another, so much so that the person becomes estranged from their own personality |
| Projection | Means of dealing with unacceptable parts of ourselves by splitting them off and attributing them to others |
| Displacement | Discharge of pent-up emotional energies on to objects or persons less threatening than the person or situation that caused them |
| Regression | Reverting to an earlier, age-inappropriate level of behaviour in order to avoid responsibility or environmental demands |

**Summary**

- Therapeutic relationships are the way in which nurses value patients as individuals and can work in partnerships with them to aid recovery.
- Nursing must maintain a balance between highly technical skills and humanistic nursing practice in order to provide the best possible care for patients.
- Therapeutic nursing is an essential component of everyday nursing practice.
- Patient-centred nursing is a style of practice that best supports the development of the nurse–patient relationship.

# References

Barber, P (1999) Caring – the nature of a therapeutic relationship. In: Perry, A (ed.) *Nursing; A Knowledge Base for Practice*, 2nd edition. Arnold, London.

Binnie, A & Titchen, A (1999) *Freedom to Practice: The Development of Patient-Centred Nursing*. Butterworth Heinemann, Oxford.

Burton, C R (2000) A description of the nursing role in stroke rehabilitation. *Journal of Advanced Nursing* 32 (1): 174–81.

Department of Health (2000) *The NHS Plan: A Plan for Investment, A Plan for Reform*. The Stationery Office, London.

Ersser, S (1997) *Nursing as a Therapeutic Activity: An Ethnography*. Avebury, Aldershot.

Freshwater, D (2003) *Counselling Skills for Nurses, Midwifes and Health Visitors*. Open University Press, Maidenhead.

Henderson, V (1980) Preserving the essence of nursing in a technological age. *Journal of Advanced Nursing* 5: 245–60.

McCormack, B (2001) *Negotiating Partnerships with Older People: A Person-centred Approach*. Ashgate Press, Aldershot.

McMahon, R & Pearson, A (1998) *Nursing as Therapy*, 2nd edition. Stanley Thornes, Cheltenham.

Mead, N & Bower, P (2000) Patient centredness: a conceptual framework and review of the empirical literature. *Social Science and Medicine* 51 (7): 1087–110.

Muetzel, P A (1988) Therapeutic nursing. In: Pearson, A (ed.) *Primary Nursing in the Burford and Oxford Development Units*. Chapman & Hall, London.

Nestel, D & Betson, C (1999) An evaluation of a communication skills workshop for dentists: cultural and clinical relevance of the patient centred interview. *British Dental Journal* 187 (7): 385–8.

NICE (2004) *The Epilepsies: The Diagnosis and Management of the Epilepsies in Adults and Children in Primary and Secondary Care*. Available at www.nice.org.uk

Orem, D (1995) *Nursing; Concepts of Practice*, 5th edition. McGraw Hill, New York.

Palmer, S, Dainbow, S & Milner, P (1996) *Counselling: The BAC Counselling Reader*. Sage, London.

Peplau, H E (1952) *Interpersonal Relations in Nursing*. Macmillan, London.

Peplau, H E (1988) *Interpersonal Relations in Nursing: A Conceptual Framework for Reference for Psychodynamic Nursing*. Macmillan, Basingstoke.

Pontin, D (1999) Primary nursing: a mode of care or a philosophy of nursing. *Journal of Advanced Nursing* 29 (3): 584–91.

Rogers, C R (1967) *On Becoming a Person*. Constable, London.

Rogers, C R (1983) *Freedom to Learn for the 80s*. Merrill, Columbus.

Royal College of Nursing (1987) *A Position Paper on Nursing*. RCN, London.

Sherwood, G D (1997) Meta-synthesis of qualitative analyses of caring: defining a therapeutic model of nursing. *Advanced Practice Nurse* 3 (1): 32–42.

Soohbany, M S (1999) Counselling as part of nursing fabric: where is the evidence? A phenomenological study using reflection on actions as a tool for framing the lived counselling experiences of nurses. *Nurse Education Today* 19: 35–40.

Thomas, L, McColl, E, Priest, J & Bond, S (1996) The Impact of primary nursing on patient satisfaction. *Nursing Times* 92 (22): 36–8.

Wright, S (1998) Facilitating therapeutic nursing and independent practice. In: McMahon, R & Pearson, A (eds) *Nursing as Therapy*, 2nd edition. Stanley Thornes, Cheltenham.

# Patient education and health promotion

8

## Learning objectives

- Describe the main principles that underpin patient education.
- Be able to apply the principles of patient education to some clinical and health educational situations.
- Describe the main principles that underpin health promotion.
- Be able to apply the principles of health promotion to some clinical and health promotional situations.

## Introduction

This chapter introduces the concepts of patient education and health promotion. These are discussed both from a theoretical perspective and in terms of application to different healthcare situations. The importance of patient education and also education for carers and families is discussed.

## Patient education

Patient education is considered to be a fundamental part of nursing care and has an important role in assisting patients in regaining independence. It is important that patients have an understanding of their condition and that they know how to manage it. This is especially true of long-term conditions where patients will be empowered to manage their condition. Hanger & Wilkinson (2001) suggest that the purpose of patient education is to provide information, reduce anxiety, change behaviour and empower patients. The aim of patient education is to improve knowledge and skills to enable patients to take control of their own condition, and this includes self-monitoring and self-management skills.

The National Institute for Health and Clinical Excellence (NICE, 2003) points out that there is insufficient evidence currently available to recommend a specific type of education or provide guidance on the setting for, or frequency of, sessions. However, they do outline some principles of good practice (Box 8.1).

Self-management of long-term conditions is playing an increasingly larger role in health care. Empowerment of patients in a number of ways, including self-management, has been a major aspect of government policy since the healthcare reforms began in 1997. More details on these reforms can be found in Chapter 13. Patient education is an essential step in supporting patient empowerment. One of the perceived advantages of patients being empowered to manage their condition is the prevention of both illness progression and potential complications (Hanger & Wilkinson, 2001). More information on the concept of patients as experts in their conditions can be found in Chapters 6 and 12.

---

### Box 8.1 Principles of good practice for patient education (adapted from NICE, 2003).

- Educational interventions should reflect established principles of adult learning.
- Education should be provided by an appropriately trained multi-disciplinary team to groups of people, unless group work is considered unsuitable for an individual.
- Sessions should be accessible to the broadest range of people, taking into account culture, ethnicity, disability and geographical issues, and could be held either in the community or at a local hospital setting.
- Educational programmes should use a variety of techniques to promote active learning (engaging individuals in the process of learning and relating the content of programmes to personal experience), adapted wherever possible to meet the different needs, personal choices and learning styles of people, and should be integrated into routine care over the longer term.

---

> **Activity**
>
> - How would you go about providing education to a patient?
> - What knowledge would you need?
> - How would you present the information?
> - How would you go about preparing for this teaching?
> - What skills would you need?
> - How would you know if the patient had understood the information?

## *The patient education process*

Webb (1997) divided the process of teaching and learning into a number of stages that can be used to build up systematic approaches to patient education. Webb (1997, p. 30–34) outlined the process of teaching and learning as follows:

- *Assessment for teaching and learning.* While this is the starting point, it is also part of the whole process. This stage involves understanding the context of the patient education. It is about good understanding and empathy, as well as beginning to plan the education in a holistic manner.
- *What does an individual need to know?* This is about comparing what the patient thinks they want to know with what the patient needs (must) to know. As a result, the agenda for the education is being set rather more from the nurse's perspective than from the patient's. It is important at this stage that clear objectives are set by the nurse.
- *Building on existing knowledge.* It is important to establish what the patient already knows. It wastes time and can be patronising if the patient has a higher level of knowledge than you assume. Likewise, a patient may have less knowledge than you expect.
- *What people want to know.* It is important to find out how much each individual patient wants to know, and this is achieved by simply asking the individual. There are some ethical considerations about how much information an individual wants, not everyone wants to know everything and there is a need to respect this wish, also it is not appropriate to withhold information from patients.
- *Preferred teaching methods and evaluation.* This will depend on the personal experience and preference of the nurse; however, the majority of patient education is one-to-one communication in some way. Most nurses use other education tools to support teaching and provide further information that can be referred to between each teaching session.

### Patient education resources

There is a vast range of educational resources available for nurses to use when teaching patients. These include information leaflets, some of which can be interactive, so that the patient has a series of exercises to go through that test whether he/she has learnt the lessons of the session, and multimedia resources, such as DVDs, again some of which are interactive. Referring patients to specific resources on the internet is also a possibility. However, many professionals also caution patients against the use of some 'non-validated' resources on the world wide web.

---

**Activity**

Consider an aspect of health that you are likely to educate a patient or group of patients about.

- What resources are available for you to use?
- Try to find as many as you can.

---

## Teaching strategies

The motivation to learn is related to the attitude people have to health and how they perceive the risk to their health. Attitudes and changing attitudes are central to the social cognition model of health, which is discussed in more detail in Chapter 1. Many studies have been carried out to examine the effectiveness of providing education to patients and also to carers and families; for example, studies that include the effectiveness of education programmes for stroke patients (Rodgers *et al.*, 1999).

One-to-one teaching has the advantage of being able to form a rapport with the patient and receive feedback from the patient. This has the advantage that the nurse has a good insight into the effectiveness of the teaching. Other teaching may be to groups, such as to a self-help group or a support group. This often involves some kind of lecture; however, it is important to supplement any presentation with the use of other resources that take advantage of encouraging the patients to use as many senses as possible. Webb (1997) suggests breaking the session up into different parts, by using a short video or group exercise.

Some teaching strategies involve the patient's family and carer as well as the patient; this, of course, needs to be done with the permission of the patient. Teaching the patient with his/her partner has the advantage that both are taking in the information, and that the partner can be involved in decisions about any changes that will affect their home life as a result of the potential changes in health behaviour.

The type of teaching required should influence the location of the teaching. For example, teaching a patient to use a hoist to get in and out of the bath might be demonstrated by using the equipment in the hospital, but the only way to make sure that the teaching has worked is to see it in action in the home. Regardless of the location of the teaching, it is important to prepare the environment so that it is conducive to learning. Privacy and the prevention of interruptions are two important principles that should be ensured. This is particularly important if the patient may be embarrassed or shocked at the information. This can stop the patient from being able to learn. Interruptions stop the flow of the teaching, and may give negative messages about the importance of the teaching to the patient. Preventing interruptions such as phone calls, or giving your bleeper to another during the teaching, are two simple examples that can improve the teaching and encourage greater success in acceptance of the information by the patient.

There is a distinction between patient education, which is largely a one-to-one or a small-group approach and constitutes a part of active health care, and health promotion, which is, in part, about a more global way of educating the population about health.

## Health promotion

Health professionals, including nurses, promote health to raise the health status of individuals and communities (Ewles & Simnett, 1997). Passive approaches, such as sales and advertising, are not health promotion as they do not necessarily raise the importance of health for the individual or the public in general. Health promotion is concerned with advancing, supporting and encouraging healthier approaches to life (Miben & Macleod-Clark, 1995). A major part of health promotion is the empowerment of patients to take control of their environment and the other factors that influence their state of health. These two aspects, improving health and taking control, of health promotion are reflected in the World Health Organisation's definition of health promotion:

> *Health promotion is the process of enabling people to increase control over, and to improve, their health* (World Health Organisation, 1984).

Health promotion, as defined by the *Ottawa Charter for Health Promotion* (World Health Organisation, 1986), refers to the 'process of enabling people to increase control over, and to improve, their health'. The implementation of this definition requires that health promotion initiatives follow a set of principles, as summarised in Table 8.1.

Health promotion has developed from health education, and the approaches used in health promotion go far wider than the traditional

**Table 8.1** Principles of health promotion. Health promotion initiatives are programmes, policies and other organised activities planned and implemented in accordance with the following principles (WHO Europe, 1998).

| Principle | Description |
| --- | --- |
| Empowering | Health promotion initiatives should enable individuals and communities to assume more power over the personal, socio-economic and environmental factors that affect their health |
| Participatory | Health promotion initiatives should involve those concerned in all stages of planning, implementation and evaluation |
| Holistic | Health promotion initiatives should foster physical, mental, social and spiritual health |
| Intersectoral | Health promotion initiatives should involve the collaboration of agencies from relevant sectors |
| Equitable | Health promotion initiatives should be guided by a concern for equity and social justice |
| Sustainable | Health promotion initiatives should bring about changes that individuals and communities can maintain once initial funding has ended |
| Multi-strategy | Health promotion initiatives should use a variety of approaches, including policy development, organisational change, community development, legislation, advocacy, education and communication, in combination with one another |

models of education (Whitehead, 2004). Although health education is still an important part of health promotion, the latter moves beyond a focus on the individual and their individual lifestyle. Ewles & Simnett (1997) use the example of putting employee health on the employment agenda as being more about political and social action and argue that it is health promotion that goes far beyond simple health education.

---

**Activity**

Can you think of health promotion campaigns that have been widely advertised through the media?

- List at least five.
- Ask your family and friends if they can think of any more.

Now consider one in particular and list what impact it has had on your health behaviour and your health beliefs.

- Did you make any changes? If so, what were they?
- Explore this further with family and friends. Did they make any changes?

## Health education programmes

There are many aspects of positive health activities in which health education programmes feature. As with different forms of health care, these can be addressed in terms of primary, secondary and tertiary health education. The major focus of primary health education is upon those individuals who are well, and is concerned with making their lives more healthy or improving their current or future health. This can be achieved in number of ways, such as education about a healthy diet, or campaigning for safer roads to reduce accidents.

Secondary health education is concerned with preventing people who have some aspect of ill health from becoming permanently or chronically ill. This might be about returning the person to full health. Examples include educating somebody who is obese, or diabetic, about a healthy or adjusted diet, or teaching somebody how to give first aid so that they can intervene after a road accident.

Tertiary health education is about maximising what Ewles & Simnett (1997) refer to as making 'the most of the remaining potential for healthy living'. If this is considered in terms of nutrition, one example would be that a patient with Crohn's disease is provided with education about the diet needed to maximise his/her quality of life. Tertiary education for individuals who have suffered an accident might include teaching them how rehabilitation can assist in reaching their best functional ability and about how to reduce the permanence of disability (Ewles & Simnett, 1997).

## Care competencies in health promotion

Ewles & Simnett (1997) identify a number of care competencies for health promotion (outlined in Box 8.2).

It is important to note that all of the factors listed in Box 8.2 are care competencies. This means that nurses must possess a satisfactory level of competence in implementing these. The first of those listed is managing, planning and evaluating. This refers to the need to be systematic in planning a health promotion project and is vital if the project is to

---

**Box 8.2 Care competencies in health promotion (Ewles & Simnett, 1997, pp. 30–31).**

- Managing, planning and evaluating
- Communicating
- Educating
- Marketing and publicising
- Facilitating and networking
- Influencing policy and practice

be effective. The second, communicating, which is discussed in detail in Chapter 6, is key to many health processes, and health promotion is no exception. Nurses must have high-quality skills in communication, whether in one-to-one encounters, group meetings or presentations, media appearances in health promotion and other situations.

While heavily related to communication, educating places emphasis upon understanding and using educational strategies in the right way, in the right circumstances and at the right time. Marketing and publicising requires particular and rare skills; for instance, a unique set of skills is required when working with the media in order to ensure that information is reported in a balanced and accurate way. Facilitating and networking skills are very important when working with groups or communities. Community workers are an excellent resource in situations where these skills are required, as they are often linked with a number of agencies and are familiar with the way that they work. Influencing policy and practice works from the macro level, such as government, for instance, to the micro level of working out the set of health promotion topics for the year in the local health centre.

## *Approaches to health promotion*

Ewles & Simnett (1997) argue that there is no single approach to health promotion and, therefore, there is a need to be flexible. However, some health professionals tend to take particular consistent approaches, depending on their professional background and codes of conduct. Ewles & Simnett (1997) propose five approaches to health promotion:

- medical
- behaviour change
- educational
- client centred
- societal.

The medical approach focuses on aiming to free the individual from medical problems, such as disease or disability. This approach stresses medical intervention(s), such as educating families about the importance of immunisations so that more children are prevented from contracting to these infections.

Behaviour change focuses on changing the attitude and behaviour of an individual or group (Whitehead, 2001). An example of this is the way in which people are encouraged to take better care of their teeth. Educational approaches focus on providing information to people so that they can make informed decisions about their health and health care. This approach implicitly includes having respect for individuals and groups to make their own decisions in an informed manner (see Chapter 6 for a further discussion of this).

Client-centred approaches focus on working with individuals to determine what they want and need to know in order to maintain and improve their health. Health promotion in this case is concerned with facilitation, that is assisting the individual to identify what concerns him/her and finding individual approaches to fulfil this concern. Societal change approaches aim to change environment, physical, social and economic factors. As a result, the focus of any change is upon the society, by making sure that health is high on the political agenda (Ewles & Simnett, 1997).

### Summary

- Patient education and health promotion are important aspects of nursing practice.
- Patient education is a fundamental part of nursing care and it has an important role in assisting patients to regain independence.
- The process of teaching and learning can be divided into a number of stages and used to build up systematic approaches to patient education.
- There are several approaches to teaching patients, including one-to-one and group teaching.
- Health promotion is about advancing, supporting and encouraging healthier approaches to life.
- A major part of health promotion is the empowerment of patients to take control of their environment and other factors that influence their state of health.
- There is no single approach to patient education or health promotion, a range of approaches needs to be considered to fit each set of circumstances.

# References

Ewles, L & Simnett, I (1997) *Promoting Health. A Practical Guide.* 3rd edition. Baillière Tindall, London.

Hanger, H C & Wilkinson, T J (2001) Stroke education: can we rise to the challenge? *Age and Aging* 30: 113–14.

Miben, J & Macleod-Clark, J (1995) Health promotion: a concept analysis. *Journal of Advanced Nursing* 22: 1158–65.

NICE (2003) Guidance on the use of patient-education models for diabetes. Available at www.nice.org.uk

Rodgers, H, Atkinson, C, Bond, S, Suddes, M, Dobson, R & Curless, R (1999) Randomised controlled trial of a comprehensive stroke education program for patients and caregivers. *Stroke* 30: 2585–91.

Webb, P (1997) *Health Promotion and Patient Education. A Professional's Guide.* Thornes, London.

Whitehead, D (2001) Health education, behavioural change and social psychology: nursing's contribution to health promotion. *Journal of Advanced Nursing* 34 (6): 822–32.

Whitehead, D (2004) Health promotion and health education. *Journal of Advanced Nursing* 47 (3): 311–20.

World Health Organisation (1984) Health promotion: a WHO discussion document on the concepts and principles. Reprinted in 1985, *Journal of the Institute of Health Education* 23: 1.

World Health Organisation (1986) *Ottawa Charter for Health Promotion.* First International Conference on Health Promotion Ottawa, 21 November 1986. WHO/HPR/HEP/95.1

World Health Organisation Europe (1998) *Health Promotion Evaluation: Recommendations to Policy-Makers Report of the WHO European Working Group on Health Promotion Evaluation.* World Health Organisation Europe, Copenhagen.

# Section 3
# Principles of Health Care Delivery

# Multi-disciplinary working

**9**

## Learning objectives

- Understand how multi-disciplinary working improves health care for patients.
- Identify the benefits of working collaboratively with other health professionals.
- Understand the use of integrated care pathways.
- Identify how patient journeys are used in clinical settings.

## Introduction

This chapter will discuss the nature of multi-disciplinary working in the delivery of health care and why this is important to patient care. Integrated care pathways and patient journeys will also be discussed to demonstrate how multi-disciplinary teams can work together to improve patient care.

## Multi-disciplinary working

Modern health care is built on a multi-disciplinary approach, and multi-disciplinary teams are an essential part of healthcare delivery (Gorman, 1998). In the increasingly complex world of modern health care, it is virtually impossible to work in isolation from other health professionals. Professionals must work together; high-quality patient care relies heavily on a healthcare team's ability to work collaboratively in delivering the best care for the patient. The aim of multi-disciplinary working is to provide consistent, high-quality health care, resulting in a seamless service across all areas of health care and social care.

Multi-disciplinary teams are groups of professionals from diverse disciplines who come together to provide comprehensive assessment, treatment and consultation for patients. Many different health professionals may be part of a multi-disciplinary team. The make up of the team is dependent on the patient and his/her individual needs. Below is a list of some of the many types of professionals who can be involved in multi-disciplinary working:

- nurse
- doctor
- physiotherapist
- occupational therapist
- speech and language therapist
- dietician
- specialist nurse
- psychologist
- chiropodist
- social worker
- health visitor

With the modernisation of the NHS, the emphasis is on a patient-centred approach to healthcare delivery, which is based around the needs of the patient; and one of the central components of patient-focused care is teamwork (Parsley & Corrigan, 1999). These professionals must work together for the benefit of the patient.

Alongside the development of the multi-disciplinary team, there is a growing expectation that all health professionals adopt new and innovative ways of working. This includes changes to their roles and blurring of role boundaries (Reveley, 2002). Multi-skilling, a concept whereby health professionals extend and expand their role, has developed. This means that many health practitioners now incorporate skills previously done by other professional groups into their roles. This improves continuity, efficiency and effectiveness of patient care (Parsley & Corrigan, 1999).

With these changes, it is even more important for health professionals to be able to work together. Quality health care can be delivered when a team of caregivers, who are well informed about the patient's needs, work collaboratively to ensure that the patient receives the right treatment, by the right person at the right time.

> **Activity**
>
> A patient's care often involves the input of many health professionals. Think about a patient you have cared for recently.
>
> - How many health professionals were involved in the patient's care?
> - Can you list them?
> - What contribution did each make to the care of the patient?
> - How did they communicate with each other to ensure continuity of care?
> - What was your role in this process?
> - How was the patient involved in this process?

One important way in which multi-disciplinary teams work together effectively is through good communication. Regular multi-disciplinary team meetings enable individual case reviews, agreed plans of care and goal setting. Multi-disciplinary team meetings take place in a number of settings, and aim to enable a consistent, agreed approach to care. This prevents unnecessary repetition and improves efficiency and effectiveness. Multi-disciplinary team meetings should include the patients and/or their carer whenever possible. It enables each health professional to comment on the assessment and progress of the patient and ensure that care is planned and coordinated in a systematic way. Coordinating care between different health professionals in this way has the additional benefit of preventing duplication of records and treatments (Johnson, 1997).

There are many examples of how collaboration by the multi-disciplinary team can lead to effectiveness and efficiency. Examples where multi-disciplinary working is particularly important include discharge planning for patients (especially those with complex needs). Without effective collaboration, this could leave the patient and carer not only dissatisfied with the service, but potentially at risk. Not only direct patient care benefits from multi-disciplinary working, practice development and service improvement also require a multi-disciplinary approach in order to be effective (McCormack *et al.*, 2005).

## The single assessment process

The single assessment process is an example of multi-disciplinary working. The single assessment process (SAP) for older people was introduced in the *National Service Framework for Older People* (Department of Health, 2001); the expectation was that it would be implemented by 2002. The purpose of SAP is to ensure that older people receive appropriate, effective and timely responses to their health and social care needs. One of the reasons this was needed was that older people frequently faced many different assessments when they accessed health and social services, including primary and secondary care and housing. Patients would often be asked the same questions many times as each different health professional carried out their own assessment of the patients. This even occurred within the same profession and there was little sharing of information between hospital and community services. The aims of SAP are presented in Box 9.1.

Most importantly, the single assessment process acknowledges that many older people have both health and social care needs, and that agencies need to work together to ensure that effective assessments are carried out and care planning is coordinated and centred around the patient. In particular, it aims to ensure that the assessment is in proportion to older people's needs, rather than filling in unnecessary paperwork and duplicate assessments. In this way, all professionals can contribute to assessments in the most effective way (Department of Health, 2002). This is reflected in the aims of multi-disciplinary working to ensure coordinated care and best use of resources.

The rest of this chapter will describe examples of how professionals collaborate to provide high-quality care for patients. The first example is concerned with the delivery of care, in the use of integrated care pathways. The second example is concerned with developing care. McCormack & Wright (1999) advocate working at a range of organisational levels, involving people working within a number of disciplines, to make a difference to the experience of people receiving health care. The patient journey process is an example of this style of collaborating.

---

**Box 9.1 Aims of the single assessment process (Department of Health, 2001).**

- Individuals are placed at the heart of assessment and care planning, and these processes are timely and in proportion to individuals' needs.
- Professionals are willing, able and confident to use their judgement.
- Care plans or statements of service delivery are routinely produced and service users receive a copy.
- Professionals contribute to assessments in the most effective way, and care coordinators are agreed in individual cases when necessary.
- Information is collected, stored and shared as effectively as possible and subject to consent.
- Professionals and agencies do not duplicate each other's assessments.

> **Activity**
>
> Find out how the single assessment process has been introduced in your area of work.
>
> - What difference does the single assessment process make to patients?
> - What difference does the single assessment process make to health professionals?

# Integrated care pathways

## *Definition*

Patient care pathways are defined by Parsley & Corrigan (1999, p. 75) as:

> *a multidisciplinary process of patient-focused care which specifies key events and assessments, occurring in a timely fashion to produce the best prescribed outcomes within the resources and activities available, for an episode of care.*

Johnson (1997) argues that pathways of care have much to offer the NHS as a tool for identifying, evaluating and then modifying processes of care delivery. They first appeared in health care in the 1980s when clinicians in the USA, looking for ways of redefining care, began to consider the use of critical pathways. The methodology actually originated in industry, particularly in engineering, in the 1950s.

In the UK, integrated care pathways (ICPs) have been developing since about 1992. They rapidly gained popularity and have been implemented across many healthcare settings, including acute, primary and private areas. It is important to note that several terms are used to describe ICPs, including 'care pathway', 'anticipated recovery pathways', 'care maps' and 'care tracts', which can sometimes make it confusing for the reader (De Luc, 2000), but they all generally refer to the same thing: integrated care pathways.

ICPs have been defined by the National Pathways Association (1996) as follows:

> *An integrated care pathway determines locally agreed, multidisciplinary practice based on guidelines and evidence where available, for a specific patient/user group. It forms all or part of the clinical record, documents the care given and facilitates the evaluation of outcomes for continuous quality improvement.*

The importance of ICPs is that they are a tool that can be used by nurses to provide appropriate care for patients. Middleton & Roberts

(2000) explain that the key elements of ICPs are that they are patient-centred, promote the use of evidence-based guidelines, reflect multi-disciplinary working and include an audit of the process and outcomes.

Similarly, Riley (1998) describes the key elements of ICPs as being:

- locally agreed
- multi-disciplinary
- based on guidelines or evidence
- for a specific patient group
- all or part of the clinical record
- a means of evaluating outcome.

## *Application*

The ICP as a tool is aimed at a defined patient group (for example, stroke patients), a group who share a beginning and end of the episode of care for the pathway (Ellis & Johnson, 1999). The beginning would be when the patients first present to healthcare services with their symptoms, and the end would be when they are discharged from health services. The patient follows the prescribed pathway of care throughout his/her treatment. ICPs are created for a group of patients with similar conditions, and all patients with that same condition follow the pathway. The purpose is to ensure that patients with the same clinical condition all receive the same, evidence-based treatment, rather than treatment based on individual clinical decisions, which may vary from clinician to clinician.

Obviously ICPs do not work in all clinical situations, Currie & Harvey (1997) see ICPs as having been developed for specific patient groups whose diagnosis and outcomes can be predicted. Johnson (2000) agrees that ICPs can be most easily applied in predictable situations, and gives examples such as planned surgery. She argues that the rationale for this is because the steps and practices delivered are usually predictable and the patient's possible route of recovery is well defined. ICPs can, however, be restrictive for patients who fall outside the normal pattern of recovery.

To give an idea of the scope of the use of ICPs, Herck *et al.* (2004) reviewed their application and found a wide range of ICPs in use. They found that 48% of ICPs existed for surgery; 26% for medical conditions such as asthma; pneumonia and stroke; 5% for rehabilitation; 4% for psychiatry and 3% for emergency medicine. There were also pathways for donor management, laboratories, radiology, palliative care, nursing education, prevention of falls and pressure sores. There were only 3.5% of ICPs for the elderly and 9% for paediatrics.

The role of the multi-disciplinary team in ICPs is paramount to their success. It is important that all members of the team, as far as is possible, are involved in assessing how patients are progressing through the clinical pathway to achieve a positive outcome. ICPs are tools that direct the multi-disciplinary team in the provision of patient-centred care, enabling interventions to be based on best available evidence during the patient's experience.

Even before the single assessment process was introduced, Johnson (2000) argued that health services were forging partnerships with social care establishments to achieve integrated working for the patient in a seamless way to enhance coordinated care across multi-agency barriers.

## *Effectiveness*

There is a consensus that ICPs provide a care delivery system that provides benefits to patient care. Ellis & Johnson (1997) suggest that many of the over 100 NHS hospitals using pathways around the UK reported positive results. Reported benefits include reduction in lengths of stay, efficient use of nursing time, reduced costs, reduced risk and reduction in readmission. Furthermore, Morris & Welsh (1996) suggest that ICPs reduce time spent on paperwork, increase patient satisfaction and the quality of information given to patients, with an improvement in clinical outcomes.

Despite the reported benefits, Wales (2003) argues that ICPs are not a solution to all healthcare issues, that their effectiveness depends on their users and that success depends on the process of implementation. Problems with ICPs can occur for a number of reasons: difficulties if a patient has a number of conditions, different routes through the healthcare system and different rates of progress for the same condition can affect the progression of a patient on a pathway.

The perception of a lack of clinical freedom and of not being able to provide individualised care may account for the variable degree of compliance with ICP documentation. Maynors-Wallis *et al.* (2004) looked at compliance in completing documentation in a study following the implementation of an ICP and found a number of reasons why staff did not comply. Staff being too busy, the intervention was not judged as being appropriate at the time, and staff forgetting to complete the paperwork were given as reasons why the pathway had been planned but was not followed.

---

**Activity**

- Have you used any integrated care pathways in your practice?
- Were they easy to use?
- What were the benefits of using them?
- How did they influence patient care?

# Patient journey

'Patient journey' is a term that is being used increasingly in health care. It is often used by healthcare organisations to explain to patients what is likely to happen to them during the treatment. However, in this chapter, patient journey refers to the process by which services for specific patient groups are appropriately redesigned to ensure that they provide patient-centred and patient-focused care. The patient journey process is a method allowing multi-disciplinary teams to work collaboratively and innovatively to modernise services for specific patient groups. The purpose of the patient journey process is to bring all of the professionals involved in the care of a specific group of patients together to develop a new patient journey, which is both patient centred and evidence-based. The aim is to improve patient care delivery and patient and carer satisfaction.

## *Patient journey process*

There are a number of variations of how this process works. The process originated to a large extent from the modernisation agency that produced improvement guides outlining the process. The process has been widely used and adapted to assist healthcare organisations to redesign their service to meet the needs of patients.

A good example of how this process can be used is the Cancer Services Collaborative (CSC) programme, which used this method to improve services for cancer patients. It recognised that mapping the patient journey is a way of trying to see health care from the patients' point of view, and a way of identifying opportunities for improvement – opportunities that might be missed if the process was only considered from a clinician's and manager's point of view.

The CSC programme describes the process of mapping the patient journey as:

- bringing together multi-disciplinary teams (MDTs) from primary, secondary and tertiary care
- revealing the complete process – rarely does a single healthcare worker know all the processes/people involved in the patient journey
- helping staff understand how complicated the systems can be for patients
- showing how many times the patient has to wait (often unnecessarily)
- showing how many visits a patient makes to hospital and how many different people a patient meets

**Table 9.1** The journey process (adapted from Campbell *et al.*, 2004).

| Stage | Description |
| --- | --- |
| Month 1: Team formation | The multi-disciplinary team is brought together<br>It is important to ensure that membership of the team includes representation from all professionals involved in the care of the patient group<br>The team agree to meet regularly and, importantly, to communicate the process to their professional colleagues whom they represent<br>A full scoping exercise is commenced to define the extent of the project |
| Month 2: Process map of current journey | The team establishes a comprehensive map of the current service provision<br>This involves describing graphically their initial picture of the current journey for the patient from the first contact with healthcare services to the discharge of the patient<br>Typically, a group of about three individuals with different backgrounds will undertake an initial mapping exercise and then this draft attempt is redrawn as necessary to encompass the experience of the entire team |
| Month 3: Patient sampling and patient interviews | One of the key aspects to the development of the patient journey is interviewing patients to gain an insight into their experiences<br>Consensus is gained about which patients are to be interviewed through a sampling exercise<br>Once the sampling has been undertaken, patients (and carers if appropriate), are interviewed by the patient journey facilitator<br>The data (interview information) are collected and analysed<br>The findings of the patient interviews are reported back to the team in terms of common themes, ensuring that confidentiality of patients is maintained |
| Month 4: Evidence | The team collects the evidence for best practice<br>Due to the multi-disciplinary nature of the team, each professional group is able to make their own unique contribution to ensure that the evidence is truly multi-professional<br>Evidence might include National Service Frameworks, Cochrane Reviews, peer-reviewed research and other examples of good practice |
| Month 5: Redesign based on patient interviews and evidence for best practice | Information from patient interviews is considered in conjunction with evidence for best practice to inform the redesign of the patient journey<br>These data support a new vision for the service; one that both the multi-disciplinary team and the patients and carers wish to see in place<br>The team agree the way forward in terms of the new patient journey and a project plan is produced |
| Month 6: New journey mapped and consensus reached | The project is brought to a close, and a consensus event is held<br>It is held to make final decisions about options for redesign and helps the team to come to agreement about these options<br>The new patient journey is finalised<br>The team then begins to implement changes identified to improve patient care delivery |

- aiding the effective planning of where to test ideas for improvements that are likely to have the most impact on achieving the project aims
- drawing out brilliant ideas, especially from staff who do not normally have the opportunity to contribute to service organisation but who really know how things work.

More information on how the process was implemented by the CSC programme can be found at http://dev.nelh.nhs.uk/nsf/cancer/about_the_guides/strategy_a.htm

The patient journey process has been used extensively at City Hospitals Sunderland NHS Foundation Trust to modernise services for patients. The trust has delivered a patient journey programme for over 6 years and has redesigned a number of patient services, including stroke, cholecystectomy, children with cerebral palsy, fertility, lung cancer, acute coronary syndrome and head injury. Design of a patient journey, outlined by Campbell *et al.* (2004), incorporates a six-month process at the end of which an action plan is produced to take the journey forward into the implementation stage. This is summarised in Table 9.1.

Most importantly, this method enables the multi-disciplinary team to work collaboratively to change working practices to benefit the needs of patients and their carers. It can lead to a comprehensive, coordinated, multi-professional service, which meets the needs of the patients and carers as well as utilising best practice guidelines to ensure optimum care.

### Summary

- Multi-disciplinary working is an effective way to deliver care for patients.
- The importance of multi-disciplinary working is reflected in the single assessment process.
- ICPs are a means of incorporating evidence-based practice within a standardised approach.
- It is not possible to use ICPs for all patient groups.
- The patient journey process is a method of redesigning services to be both patient centred and evidence-based.

# References

Campbell, S J, Gibson A F, Watson, W, Husband, G & Bremner K (2004) Comprehensive service and practice development: City Hospitals Sunderland's experience of Patient Journeys. *Practice Development in Health Care* 3 (1): 115–26.

Currie, L & Harvey, G (1997) *The Origins and Use of Care Pathways in the USA, Australia and the United Kingdom.* Report no. 15. Royal College of Nursing, Oxford.

De Luc, K (2000) Are different models of care pathways being developed? *International Journal of Health Care Quality Assurance* 13 (2): 80–86.

Department of Health (2001) *National Service Framework for Older People.* The Stationery Office, London.

Department of Health (2002) *Guidance on the Single Assessment Process for Older People.* The Stationery Office, London.

Ellis, B & Johnson, S (1997) A clinical view of pathways of care in disease management. *International Journal of Health Care Quality Assurance* 10 (2–3): 61–6.

Ellis, B & Johnson, S (1999) The care pathway: a tool to enhance clinical governance. *British Journal of Clinical Governance* 4 (2): 61–71.

Gorman, P (1998) *Managing multi-disciplinary teams in the NHS.* Kogan Page Ltd, London.

Herck, P, Vanhaecht, K & Sermeus, W (2004) Effects of clinical pathways: do they work? *Journal of Integrated Care Pathways* 8: 95–105.

Johnson, S (1997) *Pathways of Care.* Blackwell Science, Oxford.

Johnson, S (2000) Use of ICPs to manage unpredictable situations. *Professional Nurse* 16 (3): 956–8.

Maynors-Wallis, L, Rastogi, S, Virgo, N, Kosky, N, Howard, A & Brake, G (2004) Controlled evaluation of a care pathway for an acute episode of schizophrenia. *Journal of Integrated Care Pathways* 8: 106–13.

McCormack, B & Wright, J (1999) Achieving dignified care through practice development – a systematic approach. *Nursing Times Research* 4 (5): 340–52.

McCormack, B, Manley, K & Garbett, R (2005) *Practice Development in Nursing.* Blackwell Publishing, Oxford.

Middleton, S & Roberts, A (2000) *Integrated Care Pathways: A Practical Approach to Implementation.* Butterworth-Heinemann, London.

Morris, E & Welsh, R (1996) Heart to Heart. *Health Service Journal* October: 33.

National Pathways Association (1996) Available at http://www.the-npa.org.uk/

Parsley, K & Corrigan, P (1999) *Quality Improvement in Healthcare*, 2nd edition. Stanley Thornes, Cheltenham.

Reveley, S (2002) Changing Practice: the negotiated order perspective and the development of the nurse practitioner role. In: Walsh, M, Crumbie, A & Reveley S (eds) *Nurse Practitioners: Clinical Skills and Professional Issues.* Butterworth Heinemann, Oxford.

Riley, K (1998) Definition of a pathway. *National Pathways Association Newsletter* Spring: 2.

Wales, S (2003) Integrated care pathways – what are they and how can they be used? *Clinical Governance Bulletin* 4 July: 1–4.

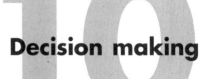

# Decision making

## Introduction

This chapter will discuss the principles underpinning the process of decision making in clinical nursing practice. This will include a discussion of the theory about decision making, and how this relates to the decisions that are made in practice. It will also include a discussion of the types of decisions that have to be made in practice and the information and other factors that affect these decisions, such as priorities of care.

Decision making is a key part of clinical practice. Nurses and other healthcare professionals make numerous decisions about patient care every day, whether in relation to direct patient care, such as the type of dressing to be used, or about indirect care, such as preparing equipment. In 1999, Thompson *et al.* identified six key areas in which nurses made decisions, these were:

- choosing between interventions
- choosing which patient will most benefit from a given intervention
- choosing the best time to carry out particular interventions
- making choices about information delivery to patients/families and colleagues
- making decisions about service delivery
- interpreting cues in the process of care.

More recently, a joint Royal College of Nursing and Department of Health funded survey (Royal College of Nursing, 2005) of nurses working in advanced and extended roles, found that 90% of respondents were regularly involved in autonomous decision making.

Decision making is an increasingly important part of nursing practice for a number of reasons. The movement towards evidence-based practice in health care (see Chapter 11) means that the best available evidence must be applied to practice. At the same time, changes to role boundaries mean that nurses are assuming increased responsibility for decision making. These changes to role boundaries have included an increasing emphasis on a multi-disciplinary approach to care delivery. As part of this, nurses have taken on more of the work traditionally undertaken by doctors. As a result of these changes, the quality of the decision making of nurses and their ability to make effective decisions has become increasingly important.

## What is decision making?

Ideally, when faced with a decision about health care, the best available evidence about the management of a condition informs the nurse and, where possible, the patient, about options that are available, together with their risks and benefits. In light of this evidence, the nurse and patient agree on a course of action and implement a plan of care. This, essentially, describes the process of decision making in an ideal world.

A number of terms are used in the literature and in practice to describe decision making. These include: clinical judgement, clinical inference, clinical reasoning, diagnostic reasoning and problem solving. To all intents and purposes, these terms are interchangeable as they describe the 'operationalisation of nursing knowledge' (Luker & Kenrick, 1992, p. 458), which is what happens in the process of decision making. That is, the nurse applies his or her knowledge to a particular situation.

There are a number of definitions of decision making. Baumann & Deber (1989, p. 1) define decision making in clinical practice as 'situations in which a choice is made from among a number of possible alternatives'. They also recognise that decision making is not a simple process, but one that often involves 'trade-offs among the values given to different outcomes' (Baumann & Deber, 1989, p. 1). That is, decisions are not always straightforward and often the nurse has to weigh up one decision against another. This may be because one decision will result in one particular outcome and another decision will result in a different one, both may be acceptable, but the outcomes have to be weighed up.

---

**Activity**

Think about a decision you made in practice recently. Think about how you came to the decision, the process you went through and what informed your decision.

- Was it straightforward and simple, or complex and difficult?
- Did you think about the outcome(s) of your decision?

---

## Decision making in nursing

The nursing profession has a linear model of analysis for decision making: the nursing process. A problem-solving approach to care, the nursing process consists of five sequential stages that are translated, in practice, into a nursing care plan (see Chapter 4 for further information about the nursing process). The nursing process can be described as an inductivist model of reasoning; that is, all available information is gathered before making any decisions, and an orderly process of data analysis is undertaken (Dowie, 1988).

## Risks in decision making

Risk taking is inherent to decision making. Nurses, in particular, are taking on new roles with decreasing supervision in an environment that is characterised by uncertainty in diagnosis, prognosis and treatment. Some areas of practice, such as emergency and intensive/critical care are recognised as 'high-risk practices' as a result of the levels of risk and uncertainty they present (Reason, 2001). However, all areas in which decisions are made involve risk taking by those making the decisions. The effects of poor decision making include the harm, or even death, of patients (Bodenham, 2005; Castledine, 2005;

Paparella, 2005; and see Chapter 14 for more information about risks and how to deal with adverse events).

The importance of nurses' ability to make effective decisions cannot be overemphasised. This means that nurses need to ensure that the information upon which they base their decisions is of good quality. This is not a simple process, however, as decisions are based on information from a variety of sources, including knowledge from evidence, practical knowledge, tacit knowledge and knowledge from reflection. It is important to remember that good decisions are made as a result of a consideration of all of the information available, which includes the wishes of the patient, clinical expertise and best evidence. There is no magic formula for this, but there are a number of tools that can assist in the process.

---

**Activity**

Think of the decisions that you make in your day-to-day work.

- Do you consider the risks as well as the benefits of making a particular decision?

Think of the risks and benefits of:

- administering a blood transfusion to a patient with impaired renal function and a haemoglobin of 8.5 g/dl.

---

# Decision making theory

Since decision making emerged as the focus of scientific enquiry in the early 1950s, a number of theories have been developed. These theories can be used to explore decision making in nursing. Essentially, they fall into three theoretical categories: descriptive, normative and pre-scriptive theories.

## Descriptive theories

Descriptive theories originate from the philosophies and professions of psychology and behavioural science (Bell *et al.*, 1988). They seek to understand *how* judgements and decisions are made in practice (Thompson & Dowding, 2002). Descriptive theories focus on the process of decision making; that is, *how* an individual arrives at a decision.

### Information-processing theories

The most frequently used descriptive theory used in nursing and midwifery is that of 'information-processing theory'. Information-processing theory (also referred to as a 'hypothetico-deductive approach') suggests that human judgement and reasoning are 'bounded' and limited to the capacity of the human memory (Newell & Simon, 1972). The theory suggests that in making decisions individuals go through a number of stages that are guided by the acquisition of cues (Elstein *et al.*, 1978):

(1)  cue acquisition, which includes technical, interactive and perceptual cues (Dowie & Elstein, 1988)
(2)  hypothesis generation
(3)  interpretation
(4)  hypothesis evaluation.

Descriptive theories emphasise heuristics, uncertainty, biases, and error in judgement and decision making. The most common way of representing heuristic knowledge is by rules of the form 'if' (condition), 'then' (action) (Clancey, 1983).

### Expertise and intuition

Expertise, as a theory for decision making, was first developed in the late 1960s (Chi *et al.*, 1988). Novice–expert theories emphasise the progress of the individual from that of a novice, to expert (Dreyfus & Dreyfus, 1980; Benner, 1984). While these theories have been widely applied to multiple professions and contexts, perhaps the most widely known in nursing is that of the model of skill acquisition (Benner, 1984) (see Chapter 16 for further details).

A popular method for explaining how expert nurses make judgements and decisions is the notion of intuition (Thomson & Dowding, 2002). Many nurses attribute at least some of their decision making to intuition, and see it as a valid and valuable part of their practice. Intuition is, however, often viewed as inferior to information processing and not regarded as 'legitimate knowledge'. However, others believe that 'intuition involves the use of sound, rational, relevant knowledge in situations that, through experience, are so familiar that the person has learned to recognise and act on appropriate patterns in the presenting problem' (Easen & Wilcockson, 1996, p. 672). Intuitive decisions are not just determined by the decision presented by a particular situation; they are also determined by the nurse making the decision. For example, an expert decision maker does not rely on protocols in his/her decision making, but has an intuitive grasp of situations, so that he/she sees the situation as a whole.

### Cognitive continuum theory

This theory views information processing and intuitive approaches as being at opposite ends of a (cognitive) continuum, with information processing at one end and intuition at the other. The basis of the theory is that nurses do not think in a purely analytical or a purely intuitive way, but in a way that it is often located at some point in between (Hamm, 1988). According to this theory, approaches adopted by the nurse are dictated by the decision he or she faces. Each decision has three dimensions:

(1) the structural complexity; for example, the number of cues present;
(2) the ambiguity of the situation; for example, how clear a diagnosis or treatment option(s) is;
(3) the way in which the information about the situation is presented; for example, subjective or objective cues.

---

**Activity**

Think about a decision you made recently in your practice. Think about how you made the decision.

- What role did information processing, your expertise and intuition play?
- Did you use all of these?
- If your information processing was included, can you identify the stages in the process you went through?
- Whereabouts on the cognitive continuum was your decision?

---

## Normative theories

Normative theories are concerned with 'what' decision or judgement was made (i.e. the outcome) and its quality, rather than the process by which the decision was made. These theories, referred to as 'rationalist' or 'decision analysis', originated from the statistical, mathematical and economic philosophies (Bell *et al.*, 1988). They aim to determine how good judgements should be made and how good outcomes should be achieved (Pruitt *et al.*, 1997). They are not concerned with how decisions are made in the 'real world', but with optimal decision making.

As indicated previously, decision making in health care is characterised by risks, uncertainty and stress. Reducing or at least identifying risks inherent to a particular decision is a central focus of normative theories. Studies that have examined errors in decision making (e.g. Reason, 2001; Vincent, 2002) show that they occur as a result of one or more of the following:

- skills-based failure, e.g. lapses in attention, distractions, interruptions, interference
- rule-based failure, e.g. in the application 'if' (condition), 'then' (action), the misapplication of good decision rules or application of bad decision rules can occur

- failure at knowledge-based level, e.g. overconfidence in the correctness of knowledge, inaccurate perceptions of abnormality, assessment clouded by recent (dissimilar) experience.

To address some of these, risk assessments, tools, scales and measurements that aim to measure and therefore reduce risks are used in health care, e.g. The Braden Scale, The Early Warning Scoring System (Thompson & Dowding, 2002).

---

**Activity**

Think about a decision you made recently in your practice, perhaps the one you used for the previous activity.

- Did you assess the risks involved in making that decision?
- How did you do this?
- Identify some of the risk assessment tools you use in your clinical practice.

Think about other decisions that you have made.

- How do you know that the decisions you make are good decisions? That is, how do you make sure that you are not overconfident in your knowledge, or distracted to the detriment of the care you provide, especially when you are very busy?

Think about some of the ways that you could avoid errors in your decision making.

- One example is collaborative decision making, list some others.

---

## Prescriptive theories

Prescriptive theories aim to improve decisions by making the process of decision making explicit (Bell *et al.*, 1988; Thompson & Dowding, 2002). Decision analysis is an example of a prescriptive model of decision making that is used in health care. It works by breaking down a decision into a number of choices, adding numerical values to each part of the decision situation (Dowie, 1993). Decision situations are usually constructed as a decision tree (Dowie, 1996) (Figure 10.1). Attached to the decision tree is the value the person attaches to each outcome (Thompson & Dowding, 2002). This improves the process of decision making by making the process and outcome explicit. Decision analysis is not appropriate for all the decisions made by nurses; however, it is very well suited to the selection of a particular treatment, for nurses and for patients, such as a choice of dressing for a wound or making

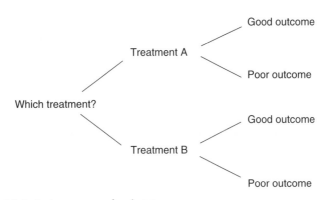

**Figure 10.1** Basic structure of a decision tree.

a decision between medical management and surgery for coronary heart disease.

### Clinical guidelines

Another example of a prescriptive model for improving clinical decisions in health care is clinical guidelines. Often referred to as protocols, because of their prescriptive nature, they aim to improve the quality and reduce variability of decisions in health care (Thompson & Dowding, 2002) (see Chapter 14 for more information on clinical guidelines).

---

**Activity**

Think of a decision you made recently in your practice.

- Did you use clinical guidelines to assist you in making the decision?
- Which clinical guideline(s) did you use?
- Can you think of other prescriptive models or tools you use in practice to assist or improve the quality of your decisions?

---

## Factors affecting decision making in practice

There are a number of factors that affect the decisions made by nurses in practice. The following is a discussion of some of these.

### *Knowledge*

Knowledge is fundamental to the definition, delineation, description and operation of a profession (Higgs & Titchen, 1995). It is essential for decision making, which is central to clinical practice. The decisions made by nurses are informed by evidence from a number of sources, which include experience (discussed earlier). The advent of National Service Frameworks (NSFs), the Commission for Health Improvement (CHI) and the National Institute for Health and Clinical Excellence (NICE), mean that evidence-based approaches to health care have become firmly established in research, professional and policy agendas. Nurses, and increasingly patients, are the vehicles through which research and evidence-based approaches to health care are applied (see Chapter 14 for further information about these and other sources of knowledge). Nurses also apply nursing theory to describe, explain, predict or prescribe nursing practice. The influence of nursing theories (see Chapter 3 for more information) on shaping nursing practice should not be forgotten.

## Tacit knowledge

Tacit knowledge is a term used to describe the knowledge that professionals use but find difficult to articulate. Tacit knowledge emerges from experience and becomes almost intuitive as practitioners act without necessarily being consciously aware of the knowledge they have. Eraut (1994) explains how tacit knowledge develops in nurses. He refers to conscious or semi-conscious pattern recognition that takes place during professional practice. Particular parts of nurses' clinical practice can become so routine that they carry them out semi-automatically. As nurses learn to perform a skill, they become increasingly less conscious of the means by which they carry this out. In such cases, the (now expert) nurses view the situation holistically, and much of their knowledge is embedded in practice. Eventually they are unable to describe the components of a skill, with any attempt to break it down into parts resulting in their inability to perform the particular skill.

## Knowledge from reflection

Reflection is an essential and enlightening skill, and the foundation of advanced practice. Reflection about thought and action provides a strategy for promoting deliberation about one's own practice within the context of particular clinical situations (Schon, 1987; Harris, 1993). It occurs when nurses contemplate past clinical situations, especially those that were confusing or particularly interesting. There are numerous theories about, and definitions of, reflective practice in the literature. Harbison (1991, p. 404), in a review of Schon's (1987) work, defined the reflective practitioner as: 'one who constantly "watches" herself in action: discovers and acknowledges the limits of her expertise, attempts to extend this . . . she is professionally mature enough to reveal uncertainty, and accept the risks inherent in all decision making'. Since reflection occurs after a particular situation, case or event, the knowledge gained can influence clinical decision making in similar (future) situations (see Chapter 16 for further discussion of reflective practice).

## *Responsibility*

Changes to the roles of nurses means that their decisions have a significant impact on healthcare outcomes and on patients' experiences. As both the extension of nurses' roles and the demand for evidence-based practice have increased, competent decisions have become imperative. The emergence of the nursing profession presents numerous implications in the realms of clinical practice (Burnard & Chapman, 1988), with the most significant perhaps its demands for increased professional responsibility 'as nurses become more accountable for their clinical decision making' (Holden, 1991, p. 398). Professional autonomy is the hallmark of professional practice (Goode, 1969; Moore, 1970; Friedson, 1971). Decision making autonomy is often equated with nurse professionalism.

---

**Activity**

Think about the decisions that you make at work and the level of responsibility you have for those decisions.

* How do you ensure that you do not practice beyond your level of responsibility, and competence?

---

## *Work culture*

Culture is:

> *a pattern of basic assumptions invented, discovered or developed by a given group ... (and) ... taught to new members as the correct way to perceive, think and feel* (Schein, 1985, p. 9).

Bower (1966) offered a more succinct definition of culture; he described the informal cultural elements of a business as 'the way we do things around here' (Bower, 1966, p. 4). This is true of decision making where 'rules' about who can and who cannot make decisions about various treatments or interventions often exist as unwritten agreements. These taken for granted and shared meanings can have a profound effect on the roles people play in decision making, for example. Many healthcare institutions, for example, remove nurses' ability to be accountable and therefore to make decisions about patient care, while others have extended their responsibilities for decision making. Given the high variability in roles performed by nurses, the variations in protocols and procedures between different settings, and the sometimes overlapping and ambiguous legislation governing the activities of medical practitioners and nurses, there is little wonder that variation in decision making occurs. Therefore in some organisations nurses will be involved in decisions that nurses in other organisations are not.

### Relationships

Many of the issues faced by nurses are not only affected by knowledge and skill development, but also by the relationships they have with others, as well as the attitudes and practices they encounter in their work. Relationships have important implications for autonomy and role. While nursing as a profession has developed, the authors are of the opinion that there are still unequal power relationships between the medical and nursing professions. The culture of healthcare organisations often contributes to unequal power relationships. Physician dominance and nurse deference have long characterised the physician–nurse relationship. In many institutions interactions between the two are carefully managed so as not to disturb the fixed hierarchy (Radcliffe, 2000). The physician–nurse game described by Stein (1967) appears, at least to some extent, to apply to current ways of working in clinical practice. While this hierarchy of power, authority and status has previously been, for the majority, invisible, recent changes to roles and role boundaries have meant that they appear increasingly as an overt conflict of interest.

### Summary

- The roles and remit of nurses' decision making about patient care are increasing, and with this comes an increase in their accountability for their decisions.
- Decision making is a complex process affected by a number of factors, not least of which are the risks and uncertainty they face in practice.
- Ensuring that good decisions are made is vital to effective patient care.
- There are a number of theories and approaches that can assist nurses in the decisions they make, both in relation to 'how' and 'what' decisions are made.

## References

Baumann, A & Deber, R (1989) *Decision Making and Problem Solving in Nursing: An Overview and Analysis of Relevant Literature.* Faculty of Nursing, University of Toronto.

Bell, D E, Raiffa, H & Tversky, A (1988) *Decision Making: Descriptive, Normative and Prescriptive Interactions.* Cambridge University Press, Cambridge.

Benner, P (1984) *From Novice to Expert: Excellence and Power in Clinical Nursing Practice.* Addison Wesley, Menlo Park, California.

Bodenham, A R (2005) Massive subcutaneous emphysema after accidental removal of an intercostal drain. *British Journal of Anaesthesia* 95 (1): 110.

Bower, M (1966) *The Will To Manage.* McGraw Hill, New York.

Burnard, P & Chapman, C (1988) *Professional and Ethical Issues in Nursing.* John Wiley & Sons, Chichester.

Castledine, G (2005) Senior nurse whose incompetence resulted in the death of a patient. *British Journal of Nursing* 14 (9): 516.

Chi, M T H, Glaser, R & Farr, M J (1988) *The Nature of Expertise.* Lawrence Erlbaum Associates Inc., Hillsdale, New Jersey.

Clancey, W J (1983) The epistemology of a rule based expert system: a framework for explanation. *Artificial Intelligence* 20: 215–51.

Dowie, J (1988) *Professional Judgement: Introductory Texts* 1–4. Open University Press, Milton Keynes. pp. 111–45.

Dowie, J (1993) Clinical decision analysis: background and introduction. In: Llewelyn H, Hopkins A (eds) *Analysing How We Reach Clinical Decisions.* Royal College of Physicians, London.

Dowie, J (1996) The research–practice gap and the role of decision analysis in closing it. *Health Care Analysis* 4: 5–18.

Dowie, J & Elstein, A (1988) Introduction to professional judgement. In: Dowie, J & Elstein, A (eds) *Professional Judgement: A Reader in Clinical Decision Making.* Cambridge University Press, Cambridge.

Dreyfus, H & Dreyfus, S (1980) A five stage model of the mental activities involved in directed skill acquisition. Unpublished study, University of California Berkley.

Easen, P & Wilcockson, J (1996). Intuition and rational decision making in professional thinking: a false dichotomy? *Journal of Advanced Nursing* 24: 667–73.

Elstein, A, Shulman, L & Sprafka, S (1978) *Medical Problem Solving: An Analysis of Clinical Reasoning.* Harvard University Press, Cambridge, Mass.

Eraut, M (1994) *Developing Professional Knowledge and Competence.* Falmer Press, London.

Friedson, E (1971) *Professions of Medicine A Study of Sociology of Applied Knowledge.* Dodd, Mead and Co., New York.

Goode, W J (1969) The theoretical limits of professionalisation. In: Etzioni, A. (ed.) *The Semi-professions and Their Organisations.* Free Press, New York. pp. 266–313.

Hamm, R M (1988) Clinical intuition and clinical analysis: expertise and the cognition continuum. In: Dowie, J & Elstein, A (eds) *Professional Judgement: A Reader in Clinical Decision Making.* Cambridge University Press, Cambridge.

Harbison, J (1991) Clinical decision making in nursing. *Journal of Advanced Nursing* 16: 404–7.

Harris, J B (1993) New expectations for professional competence. In: Curry, L & Wergin, J (eds) *Educating Professionals: Responding to the New Expectations of Competence and Accountability.* Josey Bass, San Francisco. pp. 17–22.

Higgs, J & Titchen, A (1995) Propositional, professional and personal knowledge in clinical reasoning. In: Higgs, J & Jones, M (eds) *Clinical Reasoning in the Health Professions.* Butterworth Heinemann, London.

Holden, R J (1991) Responsibility and autonomous nursing practice. *Journal of Advanced Nursing* 16 (4): 398–403.

Luker, K A & Kenrick, M (1992) An exploratory study of the sources of influence on the clinical decisions of community nurses. *Journal of Advanced Nursing* 17: 457–66.

Moore, W (1970) *The Professions: Roles and Rules.* Russell Sage Foundation, New York.

Newell, A & Simon, H A (1972) *Human Problem Solving.* Prentice Hall, Englewood Cliffs, New Jersey.

Paparella, S (2005) Inadvertent attachment of a blood pressure device to a needleless IV 'Y-site': surprising, fatal connections. *Journal of Emergency Nursing* 31 (2): 180–82.

Pruitt, J S, Cannon-Bowers, J A & Salas, E (1997) In search of naturalistic decisions. In: Flin, R, Salas, E, Strub, M & Martin, L (eds) *Decision Making Under Stress: Emerging Themes and Applications.* Ashgate Publishing, Aldershot, England.

Radcliffe, M (2000). Doctors and nurses: new game, same result. *British Medical Journal* 320 (7241): 1085.

Reason, J (2001) Understanding adverse events: the human factor. In: Vincent, C (ed.) *Clinical Risk Management.* British Medical Journal Books, London.

Royal College of Nursing (2005) *Maxi Nurses: Nurses Working In Advanced And Extended Roles Promoting And Developing Patient-Centered Health.* RCN, London.

Schein, E H (1985) *Organisational Culture and Leadership.* Jossey-Bass, San Francisco.

Schon, D A (1987) *Educating the Reflective Practitioner.* Jossey Bass, San Francisco.

Stein, L I (1967) The doctor–nurse game. *Archives of General Psychiatry* 16: 699–703.

Thompson, C, McCaughan, D, Cullum, N, Sheldon, T, Thompson, D & Mulhall, A (1999) *Nurses' Use Of Research Information In Clinical Decision Making: A Descriptive and Analytical Study.* Available at http://www.york.ac.uk/health sciences/centres/evidence/decrpt.pdf

Thompson, C & Dowding, D (2002) *Clinical Decision Making and Judgement in Nursing.* Churchill Livingstone, London.

Vincent, C (2002) Enhancing patient safety. In: Vincent, C (ed.) *Clinical Risk Management.* British Medical Journal Books, London.

# Evidence-based practice

---

## Learning objectives

- Understand what evidence-based practice is and what it means for healthcare delivery.
- Identify the types of evidence that inform best practice.
- Understand the importance of implementing evidence-based practice.
- Understand the principles of finding, appraising and applying evidence.
- Be familiar with the range of barriers and resources to implementing evidence-based practice.
- Understand the importance of evaluating the implementation of evidence-based practice.

---

## Introduction

In this chapter the principles of evidence-based practice (EBP) will be defined, and we will discuss the importance of the 'finding, appraising and applying' process of evidence-based practice, the barriers that affect its implementation in clinical practice, the systems that are in place to support it, and the importance of evaluating its implementation.

# What is evidence-based practice?

Evidence-based practice (EBP) has become a central issue in modern health and social care. In the UK the movement towards EBP has been supported by the government and is regarded as an essential part of the modern health service (Department of Health, 1998). Evidence-based practice ensures that the care that is delivered is the most effective. This means that care should be based on the best available evidence, not on tradition or because it has always been done that way. By doing this, care that is ineffective, inappropriate, expensive or potentially dangerous is reduced or eliminated.

Developments in health care in most Westernised countries over the past 10 years have been driven by a desire to improve effectiveness, efficiency and health outcomes for patients. The notion of 'best practice' relates closely to this focus, and is being linked increasingly to the need to base practice on the best-available evidence. Its origins, which extend back to the mid-nineteenth century, grew out of concerns about health-care interventions not being proven or evaluated.

# Definitions of evidence-based practice

Several terms are used to describe clinical practice that is based on best evidence, they are: evidence-based practice, evidence-based health care and evidence-based medicine. Essentially they all refer to the same process, but focus on different areas; for example, evidence-based medicine is focused on the medical profession, in contrast to evidence-based health care, which addresses the broader aspects of care delivery.

Probably the most widely used definition is that of Sackett and his colleagues (Sackett *et al.*, 1996, p. 71), who refer to evidence-based medicine, and state:

> *Evidence based medicine is the conscientious, explicit, and judicious use of current best evidence in making decisions about the care of individual patients. The practice of evidence based medicine means integrating individual clinical expertise with the best available external clinical evidence from systematic research.*

Evidence-based practice is all encompassing. It recognises the need for health care to be individualised and responsive to changing situations in order to achieve effective and efficient practice that meets the needs of patients. Effective practice is about 'what' care practitioners deliver and efficient practice is about 'how' practitioners deliver that care. McKibbon (1998, p. 396) defined evidence-based practice as:

*. . . an approach to health care wherein health professionals use the best evidence possible, i.e. the most appropriate information available, to make clinical decisions for individual patients. EBP values, enhances and builds on clinical expertise, knowledge of disease mechanisms, and pathophysiology. It involves complex and conscientious decision-making based not only on the available evidence but also on patient characteristics, situations, and preferences.*

## Why should practice be evidence-based?

It is important that nurses not only know 'how' to do something, but also to understand 'why' it is being done. In this way evidence-based practice is linked with clinical effectiveness: doing the right thing in the right way and at the right time for the right patient (Royal College of Nursing, 1996) (see Chapter 15 for more information about clinical effectiveness). For this reason, nurses need to deliver health care that is both evidence-based and patient centred. The National Health Service (NHS) Plan (Department of Health, 2000) calls for improvement in service provision, better use of research and the delivery of evidence-based health care.

The movement towards 'research and evidence-based practice' in health care is based, at its simplest, on the argument that professionals have a moral responsibility to practise in ways that are underpinned by the best evidence available and that are improved by building that evidence base. Ideally, the best available evidence about the management of a condition informs the practitioner, and the patient (where possible), about options that are available, together with their risks and benefits. This is embedded in the Nursing and Midwifery Council's *Code of Professional Conduct* (2002) section 6.5, which states:

*As a registered nurse, midwife or health visitor, you must maintain your professional knowledge and competence. You have a responsibility to deliver care based on current evidence, best practice and, where applicable, validated research when it is available.*

The government's Clinical Governance agenda also includes the requirement that 'Evidence-based practice (should be) in day to day use with the infrastructure to support it' (Secretary of State for Health, 1997).

> *Remember:*
> *Evidence-based practice is not about*
> *just doing things right, or doing the right things,*
> *but doing the right things right!*

# What is evidence?

It is important to consider what constitutes best evidence. Evidence itself may be defined as 'ground for belief, testimony or facts tending to prove or disprove any conclusion' (Simpson & Weiner, 1994). There are a number of different types of evidence that can be used to inform EBP.

## Evidence from research

Research is 'the attempt to derive generalisable new knowledge by addressing clearly defined questions with systematic and rigorous methods' (Department of Health, 2003, p. 4). It is a systematic search for information, a process of enquiry and investigation, the general purpose of which is to contribute to the evidence base that shapes and guides practice. In health care there is an assumption that 'science'-based evidence will tell us the most effective approaches to care delivery. This evidence comes from quantitative research studies, in particular the randomised controlled trial (RCT), which is seen as the 'gold standard' in evidence of effectiveness. Randomised control trials try to eliminate experimental bias as much as is possible. Patients are randomly allocated to either a trial group or a control group, and differences in health outcomes against set criteria are measured and, where applicable, attributed to the medical intervention. Double-blind RCTs are conducted in much the same as RCTs, but to eliminate bias further, the clinicians are unaware of which group patients belong to. It is important to remember that qualitative research also provides evidence that is relevant to health care and is used increasingly to provide information about patient views and experiences of health care.

The way evidence is used to inform practice is, to some extent, affected by the quality and availability of evidence, and by the method(s) used to carry out the research. This is reflected in the hierarchy of evidence, which provides guidelines for interpreting the strength of the evidence provided, on a given topic. Figure 11.1 shows systematic reviews and meta-analysis at the top of the hierarchy of evidence, indicating that they are important sources of evidence. They are also referred to in the literature (for example see NICE Guidance: www.NICE.org.uk) as category I (one) evidence. A systematic review attempts to synthesise all of the available evidence on a particular problem or condition. This provides an overview from which conclusions can be drawn in an attempt to identify the most appropriate action to take.

While the RCT is recognised as the 'gold standard' in evidence of effectiveness, health professionals and patients face questions about health care that cannot always be answered by this method of enquiry.

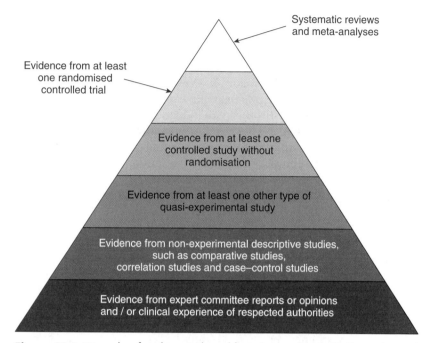

**Figure 11.1** Hierarchy of evidence (adapted from Agency for Health Care Policy and Research, 1992).

Each patient is an individual with physical, social and emotional needs. Issues in health care are not all to do with medical and technical interventions or treatments; they are also to do with relationships, practices, attitudes and values. Increasingly, evidence and knowledge from patients and their carers about their healthcare experience(s) and the management of their condition is being used to inform care delivery. In recognising this, it is important to use the most appropriate evidence for the clinical practice situation and, therefore, to use evidence from the full range of the hierarchy to best achieve EBP.

---

**Activity**

- Are you familiar with the research-based evidence that underpins the health care you provide?
- What sort of research is most common in supporting your practice?
- How can you be sure that the care you provide is evidence-based?

---

## Expertise as evidence

A popular method for explaining how expert nurses make judgements and decisions is that they develop professional expertise through their experience (Thomson & Dowding, 2002). There is, however, debate about whether practical expertise is 'evidence'. This debate is centred on what constitutes 'real' evidence, which, as indicated above, is that derived from research findings that have been validated through rigorous, quantitative research. Closs (2003) for example, argues that although clinical expertise is essential to the delivery of high-quality care, it does not constitute evidence *per se*. Part of the reason for her view is the misconception that experience will always lead to excellence in practice. Closs's (2003) view is supported by Benner's (1984) earlier work on the development of the expert nurse. Benner (1984, p. 178) refers to experience in terms of years of practice, and also includes a definition of experience which 'does not necessarily refer to longevity and/or length of time in a position'. In support of this, there are situations in which, for a variety of reasons, nurses do not learn from experience. Consequently, for some nurses, 20 years' experience is 20 years of gaining more practical knowledge, while for others it is 1 year's experience repeated 20 times.

Others take a different view about evidence from professional experience. Eraut (1994) describes this form of evidence as 'practical knowledge' that is embedded in practice. He refers to intuition and tacit knowledge, both of which, he states, are difficult to articulate. There are some who consider that scientific methods of reasoning are 'real thinking' and that intuition and tacit knowledge are not 'legitimate knowledge' (e.g. Benner, 1984). However, both should be recognised as valuable elements of knowledge. Experienced nurses, for example, have included 'gut feelings' when they list the different components that influence their practice. For some nurses 'gut feelings' refer to a 'falling out of pattern' in the signs and symptoms of the patient, while for others it means an 'intuitive' feeling. The experience of making an intuitive professional decision is not only disconcerting for a number of practitioners but, at least for some, is also considered to be in some way unprofessional, with intuitive judgements being compared unfavourably with 'rational', 'scientific', professional practice.

Easen & Wilcockson (1996) believe that the debate about intuition seems to stem from the mistaken belief that intuition is an irrational process. While intuition may be seen as an irrational process, the basis of the intuitive decision need not be so. The nature of the knowledge and pattern recognition used by the practitioner is based on knowledge and experience (see Chapter 10 for further discussion of expertise and intuition and tacit knowledge).

Practical knowledge is not based purely on science; it is gained from experiencing a range of situations. It is characterised by a complex combination of doing and thinking which cannot be separated into theoretical and practical components. Theoretical knowledge has to be applied in the practical situation, i.e. something learnt in the classroom only becomes practical knowledge when it is experienced in real life. Moore (1970), in support of this view, identifies two major components of professional expertise: (1) the substantive field of knowledge, and (2) the technique of applying that knowledge. In nursing we must differentiate between knowing how to do something and 'acting knowledge'. The former is simply a method of doing something, focused solely on the task, the latter goes beyond knowing 'how' to knowing 'what to do when', 'where', by 'whom' and 'why'.

Recent research has shown that nurses draw upon this practical knowledge (Thompson *et al.*, 2001) more frequently than formal sources of knowledge, such as published research reports (Gerrish & Clayton, 2004). Indeed, there is increasing opinion that the overriding emphasis of EBP on RCTs undermines the value of the clinician and ignores the social and psychological aspects of health care (Williams & Garner, 2002). Further, where there is a lack of empirical or research-based evidence, expertise is used to inform practice. This expertise comes both from healthcare professionals and from patients, who are taking an increasingly active role in the development of health care.

---

**Activity**

Do you think evidence from experience is real evidence?

- Think about your answer and why you believe this.
- If you don't believe this, what do you do when there is no research-based evidence?

Can you recall using intuition or tacit knowledge in the decisions you make about care?

- What was that like?
- How did others react?
- Could you explain the basis of your decision/care?

Identify a particular part of your clinical practice that you performed recently, for example a wound dressing, observations or health education. Consider the following:

- Do you know of any evidence to support your actions?
- What type of evidence is it?
- Where does it fit in the hierarchy of evidence?

- Where do you find evidence to support your actions if you need to?

## Finding–appraising–applying evidence

It is important that clinical practice is based on current best evidence. The use of evidence in practice requires a three-stage process of information gathering, appraisal and application. This is by no means a linear process, but a dynamic, interactive ongoing cycle in which evidence is continually sought, evaluated and used to inform practice (Figure 11.2).

### *Finding evidence*

Once an area of need in practice has been identified, the first step in the process of implementing EBP is the identification of new evidence to inform practice. There are an increasing number of resources available from which evidence can be found. As these resources increase, so does the need for nurses to acquire and develop the skills to search effectively. This is important in order that nurses can contribute to the development of evidence-based clinical practice, as well as developing policies and evaluating practice.

#### Journals and databases

One valuable source of research literature is journals and journal articles. Many of these contain editorials, case studies and reports as well as research. It has been estimated that 2 million articles are published in 20,000 biomedical journals every year. This would form a stack 500 m high. 'To keep up to date with current literature a (nurse) would need to read and appraise 19 original articles a day – every day' (Davidoff *et al.*, 1995, p. 1085). To address this, there are a number of electronic databases, in addition to CINAHL and MEDLINE®, that can be used to locate research relating to a particular area. These increasingly offer full text articles online. The websites below are recognised as valuable resources in searching for best evidence. Some of these sites include journals and journal articles, while others provide systematic reviews, policy documents, guidelines and national service frameworks. Clinical practice guidelines consist of statements that are systematically

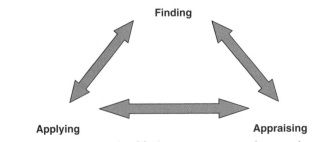

Finding

Applying                    Appraising

**Figure 11.2** The dynamic cycle of finding–appraising–applying evidence.

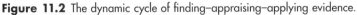

developed to assist practitioner and patient decisions about appropriate health care for specific clinical conditions. An increasing number of well-constructed, practical and evidence-based guidelines are being developed. National Service Frameworks (NSFs) set national service standards, define models for a specific service or care group, and suggest strategies to support their implementation. They identify key interventions and set measurable goals to be achieved within an agreed time scale. NSFs are long-term strategies for improving specific areas of care. They are developed as a result of an extensive consultation exercise with leading practitioners, researchers, patients and carers (see Chapter 14 for further discussion of clinical guidelines and NSFs).

## Valuable resources for finding evidence

*National Communicating Centre for NHS Service Delivery and Organisation National Research and Development Programme*
This programme was launched in March 2000 to produce and promote the application of best evidence about how the organisation and delivery of services can be improved to increase the quality of patient care, ensure better outcomes and contribute to improve health in the wider community.

*The Department of Health (DH)*
http://www.dh.gov.uk

Responsible for setting health and social care policy in England, the Department of Health sets standards and guidelines and National Service Frameworks (NSFs) for care across all areas of the NHS, social care and public health. The Department also provides some guidance on the implementation of these standards, guidelines and NSFs.

*National Electronic Library for Health (NeLH)*
http://www.nelh.nhs.uk/

An official NHS site, the NeLH provides healthcare professionals with best evidence support for the delivery of evidence-based health care. It has links to a number of relevant organisations as well as to specialist and health libraries and to a guidelines finder, which provides an index to over 1200 UK guidelines with links to downloadable versions.

*Cochrane Library and Cochrane Database of Systematic Reviews*
http://www.nelh.nhs.uk/cochrane.asp

The Cochrane Library is an electronic publication designed to supply high-quality evidence to inform people providing and receiving care, and those responsible for research, teaching, funding and administration at all levels. The Database of Systematic Reviews is a growing collection of systematic reviews of the effects of health care.

*Evidence-Based Medicine Reviews*
http://www.ovid.com/site/catalog/DataBase/904.jsp

Evidence-Based Medicine Reviews (EBMR) is an electronic information resource which combines three EBM sources into a single, fully searchable database with links to MEDLINE® and Ovid full-text journals.

*National Health Service's Centre for Reviews and Dissemination (NHS CRD)*
http://www.york.ac.uk/inst/crd/

Provides research-based information about the effects of interventions used in health and social care.

*The Royal College of Nursing (RCN)*
http://www.rcn.org.uk/

As part of its clinical effectiveness work, the RCN develops national nurse-led guidelines. The College is also involved in informing the development of other guidelines, providing a nursing perspective through membership of steering groups. The RCN website provides links to partner organisations.

**Other resources**
As well as the resources above, there are a number of other means of finding evidence. Many research projects that are carried out are not published in journals, but as reports. These can be useful sources of information, but it should be remembered that they have not been through the rigorous review process of journals and therefore may not be of the same standard. This can also be true for what is known as the 'grey' literature, which includes unpublished research, pamphlets and circulars. Although often not up to date with the most recent evidence, books can provide a useful background to an area of interest.

**Searching the literature**
Before starting to search for evidence, it is important that the area of interest is clearly defined. This will save time and make the search more effective. A helpful way of refining the area of interest is to:

Start with individual broad concepts
and combine them together
gradually narrowing your
search down
as you
go

For example, an interest in heart conditions, might be refined to an interest in heart rhythms, which might be refined further to adults with tachycardia, and even further to the effects of digoxin on adults with tachycardia. Once the area of interest has been clearly defined, another helpful method is to break the question down into clearly defined concepts using the PICO acronym (Ask an Expert, 2002). The acronym is made up as follows:

- Patients/Problem (e.g. adults with tachycardia)
- Intervention/Exposure (e.g. digoxin)
- Comparisons (e.g. no digoxin)
- Outcomes (e.g. reduced incidence of tachycardia)

These concepts can then be used to carry out a search of the literature. This can be done electronically or manually. Electronic searching provides access to a wide range of resources at one time, but can be intimidating as each database is different and requires particular techniques to be used. It is important not to be put off by this, however, as there are a number of key techniques that are common to many databases. Manual searching is an important part of finding evidence, as some evidence is not yet included in electronic form, especially the most recent editions of journals. Journal indices, tables of contents and reference lists are good places to start when searching this way. The best way to learn how to search the literature using these resources is by doing just that, using them. The best place to start is at a library or local research department, where trained staff can assist in how to search and provide information about the most effective use of these sources, as well as providing information about training courses.

## *Appraising evidence*

It is important that the quality of the evidence used to inform practice is assessed and that it is not simply accepted as best evidence. Evidence from research findings needs to be appraised critically by individuals with the knowledge and skills to do so. Critical appraisal is 'the process of assessing and interpreting evidence by systematically considering its validity, results and relevance' (Parkes *et al.*, 2001, p. 10). There are numerous checklists that can be used to appraise evidence critically. While critical appraisal techniques and tools vary according to the type of evidence being reviewed, i.e. the type of study that was conducted, there are three questions that appear common to all quantitative studies:

- Are the results of the study valid? Validity relates to the truth of the findings in the real world. If the methods used do not relate to what happens in the real world, they are not valid and nor are any results. For example, if a drug is tested only on patients with the most severe form of asthma, or excludes patients who have impaired renal function, we cannot use these results directly to determine the treatment of patients with less severe asthma or patients with impaired renal function.

- What are the results of the study and are they reliable? It is important to establish that the results of the study did not occur by chance. That is, it is important to determine that if we repeated the research, and measured the same outcomes, we would find the same results.
- Do the results apply to the local situation? However strong the results of a study, its application at a local level has to be considered. This is, of course, unless it has been carried out to inform national policy and guidance for practice. Decisions to implement new evidence are dependent upon a range of factors, including financial and other resources, the skills of staff and organisational policy.

Critical appraisal methods and tools for qualitative research are less developed than those for quantitative research. Despite this, it is important that these studies are subject to critical appraisal and that the following issues are addressed:

- Rigour: has a thorough and appropriate approach been applied to key research methods in the study?
- Credibility: are the findings well presented and meaningful?
- Relevance: how useful are the findings to you and your organisation?

Due to the variation in the amount of research available, differences in professional opinion and in local requirements about clinical practice, it is often difficult to appraise evidence and to determine what is best. There are, however, a number of organisations that offer guidance, including critical appraisal tools.

*Critical Appraisal Skills Programme (CASP)*
http://www.phru.nhs.uk/casp/

*Users Guide for Evidence-Based Practice*
www.cche.net.usersguides/main.asp

*CONSORT*
http://www.consort-statement.org/

The CONSORT statement for improving the quality of reporting of randomised controlled trials.

*Health Technology Assessment Reports*
http://www.hta.nhsweb.nhs.uk/ProjectData/3_publication_listings_ALL.asp

This resource at the Wessex Institute for Research and Development contains abstracts for the completed reviews from the National Health Service Health Technology Assessment Programme.

*AGREE (Appraisal of Guidelines Research and Evaluation)*
http://www.agreecollaboration.org/

AGREE is an international collaboration of researchers and policy makers who seek to improve the quality and effectiveness of clinical practice guidelines.

*Cochrane Collaboration Handbook*
http://www.cochrane.org/resources/handbook/

The Cochrane Collaboration's handbook is its main working document. It provides practical guidance for developing and conducting Cochrane Systematic Reviews.

## Applying evidence

EBP does not just happen; someone or something has to make it happen. The use of evidence in professional nursing practice requires interpretation and application by the nurse using the evidence in practice. In order that EBP is promoted, it is essential to understand the strategies that facilitate the effective introduction and application of research. The factors affecting the implementation of EBP are a combination of available evidence and the development of skills, as well as wider factors such as relationships, practices, attitudes and values.

Evidence should not only inform practice, it should change practice. Whatever the area identified, whether it is a specific clinical issue or a broader matter about care delivery, and however large or small the difference between current and new practice, there will be a need to change practice or policy. There are a number of different levels of change required in clinical practice in order that EBP is implemented:

- a change that needs to be addressed immediately
- a change that can be implemented immediately
- a change that needs to be addressed by a ward or department team
- a change that needs addressing by the organisation as a whole.

The processes involved in the implementation of EBP include a range of strategies and methods. There is no single method or approach, and their uses will be determined by the requirements of the change required and the particular situation. Some knowledge of change processes is an important aspect to the successful implementation of EBP (these are discussed in Chapter 15). Many of the approaches to change found in the literature give the impression that change is simple. In practice, however, implementing change is often a complex process. It requires practitioners to change their practice when it is no longer what is best for the patient, for example when new evidence becomes available.

# Barriers to achieving evidence-based practice in nursing

## Resistance to change

Barriers to achieving EBP come from a number of factors, which include a reluctance to change existing practice(s), often based on tradition and which have 'always been done that way'. Avoidance of change can often result in the development of ritualistic practices. Given the complexity of change, there is no single method that could be reliably expected to change practice in all circumstances and settings. It is worth considering that a combination of these approaches can help to compensate for the limitations of each. There are guiding principles that can be adapted to the implementation of EBP in a variety of situations. The NHS Centre for Reviews and Dissemination's (1999) findings about helpful approaches to implementing EBP are summarised in Box 11.1.

---

**Box 11.1 Helpful approaches to implementing evidence-based practice (NHS Centre for Reviews and Dissemination, 1999).**

- Be clear about the proposed change, why it is necessary, what do you hope to achieve (what are your anticipated outcomes?) and what evidence supports it?
- How prepared are other health professionals to implement the proposed change and how you are going to present your proposal to them?
- Identify and, where possible, include representatives from all groups and individuals involved in, affected by or influencing the proposed change(s) in practice; a wide range of people may be involved, including health professionals, managers, policy makers, researchers and the public.
- Ensure that this group feeds information and plans back to their colleagues so that those not directly involved are provided with the opportunity to discuss and influence the change. Identify any potential barriers to the change and consider how you might address these.
- Identify any factors that may support the change, including individuals and resources.
- Remember, most changes are effective under some circumstances; none are effective under all circumstances.

---

> **Activity**
>
> Think about the people that you work with and how they might react to evidence-based practice.
>
> - Who might be in favour of clinical practice not founded in evidence?
> - Why?

## The nature of evidence about nursing practice

While there has been a considerable increase over the past decade in the amount of research that examines nursing practice, there is relatively little research that connects nursing care directly with patient outcomes. This has been as a result of the difficulty in making links between nursing care and patient outcomes, as well as a tendency towards small scale, local studies, that focus on local need(s). However, as the role of nurses continues to develop, it is likely that it will become easier to link nursing interventions with patient outcomes and therefore possible to increase the evidence base for nursing practice.

## The publication of evidence

Nurses' tendency to draw upon practical knowledge from their colleagues (Thompson *et al.*, 2001) more than formal sources of knowledge, such as published research (Gerrish & Clayton, 2004), occurs in part because of the way that research is published. It is often published in academic journals, in a style that is not particularly accessible to nurses and which, as a result, they tend not to read (McCaughan *et al.*, 2002).

## Critical appraisal skills

While willing to use research, many nurses may lack the skill and time to appraise it critically. While critical appraisal skills training is increasingly a part of the nursing curriculum, the regular application of these skills is required in order that they are maintained. Critical appraisal requires considerable knowledge about the research process and can be very time consuming. Arguably, a focus on clinical skills and patient care at the outset of their career takes precedence over these skills, which then have to be re-learnt.

# Resources to aid the implementation of evidence-based practice

In the UK, the application of best evidence is promoted through the development and dissemination of Clinical Guidelines and National

Service Frameworks. The implementation of guidelines and NSFs helps practitioners assimilate, evaluate and implement evidence and consensus on best current practice and provides a method of bridging the gap between evidence and everyday practice (SIGN, 1999). The implication is that implementing guidelines and NSFs will lead to changes in practice that improve patient care and outcomes. In addition to this there are a number of organisations that offer guidance on the implementation of evidence into practice:

*School of Health and Related Research [SchHARR]*
http://www.shef.ac.uk/scharr/ir/guidelin.html

This lists of a number of guidelines available in full-text from the world wide web.

*National Institute for Health and Clinical Excellence [NICE]*
http://www.nice.org.uk/page.aspx?o=implementation

Contains resources for people who have responsibility for implementing guidelines.

*Department of Health*
http://www.dh.gov.uk/PolicyAndGuidance/HealthAndSocialCar
Topics/fs/en#4935897

Provides national standards for a number of care groups.

## Evaluating a change to practice

It is vital that any change to clinical practice is evaluated. This is in order to establish:

- if the change has worked, i.e. has it taken place? and
- if it has had the desired outcome, i.e. have the objectives of the change, and therefore an improvement in care, been met?

The success of the change can be relatively easy to evaluate if there is a measurable outcome, such as the documentation of respiratory rate as a routine observation for all patients, for example. In nursing, however, the desired outcome of a change is often more complex, and there may not be a measurable outcome that can be attributed directly to the change. In these cases it may be necessary to undertake a more comprehensive evaluation of the change. This can be a complex process and may require the involvement of specially trained staff. Ideally, when planning to implement a change to current practice it is advisable that a representative from the research or audit department is included. That way they will better understand the proposed change(s) and will be more able to assist in the evaluation.

### Summary

- Evidence-based practice is an attempt to move away from traditional, ritualistic practice and is a move towards ensuring that patients receive the best possible care.
- It is a dynamic, interactive, ongoing cycle in which evidence is continually sought, evaluated and applied in order that clinical practice is based on best evidence.
- Evidence-based practice can be achieved by using both evidence from research and knowledge that can be found from a range of sources.
- Implementing evidence-based practice involves a continuous process of finding, appraising and applying evidence.
- There are a number of barriers and aids to implementing evidence-based practice.
- It is important to remember that any change to practice should be evaluated.

## References

Agency for Health Care Policy and Research (1992) *Acute Pain Management: Operative or Medical Procedures and Trauma.* Department of Health and Human Services, Public Health Service, Rockville, MD, USA.

Ask an Expert (2002) Popping the PICO Question in research and evidence based practice. *Applied Nursing Research* 15: 197–8.

Benner, P (1984) *From Novice to Expert Excellence And Power In Clinical Nursing Practice.* Addison Wesley, Menlo Park, California.

Closs, S J (2003) Evidence and community-based nursing practice. In: Bryer, R & Griffiths, J (eds) *Practice Development in Community Nursing.* Arnold, London. pp. 33–56.

Davidoff, F, Haynes, B, Sackett, D & Smith, R (1995) Evidence-based medicine. *British Medical Journal* 310: 1085–6.

Department of Health (1998) *A First Class Service.* The Stationery Office, London.

Department of Health (2000) *The NHS Plan: a Plan for Investment, a Plan for Reform.* Stationery Office, London.

Department of Health (2003) *Draft Research Governance Framework for Health and Social Care*, 2nd edition. The Stationery Office, London.

Easen, P & Wilcockson, J (1996) Intuition and rational decision making in professional thinking: a false dichotomy? *Journal of Advanced Nursing* 24: 667–73.

Eraut, M (1994) *Developing Professional Knowledge and Competence.* Falmer Press, London.

Gerrish, K & Clayton, J (2004) Promoting evidence-based practice: an organisational approach. *Journal of Nursing Management* 12: 114–23.

McCaughan, D, Thompson, C, Cullum, N, Sheldon, T & Thompson, D (2002) Acute care nurses' perceptions of barriers to using research information in clinical decision making. *Journal of Advanced Nursing* 39 (1): 46–60.

McKibbon, K A (1998). Evidence based practice. *Bulletin of the Medical Library Association* 86 (3): 396–401.

Moore, W (1970) *The Professions: Roles and Rules.* Russell Sage Foundation, New York.

NHS Centre for Reviews and Dissemination (1999) *Effective Health Care: Getting Evidence into Practice* 5 (1): 1–16. NHS CRD, University of York, UK. Available at http://www.york.ac.uk/inst/crd/ehc51.pdf

Nursing and Midwifery Council (2002) *Code of Professional Conduct.* NMC, London.

Royal College of Nursing (1996) *Clinical Effectiveness A Royal College of Nursing Guide.* RCN, London.

Sackett, D L, Rosenberg, W M C, Muir Gray, J A, Haynes, R B & Richardson, W S (1996) Evidence based practice: What it is and what it isn't. *British Medical Journal* 312 (7023): 71–2.

Schon, D A (1987) *Educating the Reflective Practitioner.* Jossey Bass, San Francisco, California.

Secretary of State for Health (1997) *The New NHS: Modern, Dependable.* The Stationery Office, London.

SIGN (1999) *SIGN Guidelines: An Introduction to SIGN Methodology for the Development of Evidence Based Clinical Guidelines.* Publication No. 39. SIGN, Edinburgh.

Simpson, J A & Weiner, E S (eds) (1994) *Oxford English Dictionary,* 2nd edition. Oxford University Press, Oxford.

Thompson, C & Dowding, D (2002) *Clinical Decision Making and Judgement in Nursing.* Churchill Livingstone, London.

Thompson, C, McCaughan, D, Cullum, N, Sheldon, T, Mullhall, A & Thompson, D (2001) The accessibility of research-based knowledge for nurses in United Kingdom acute care settings. *Journal of Advanced Nursing* 36 (1): 11–22.

Williams, D D R & Garner, J (2002) The case against 'the evidence': a different perspective on evidence-based medicine. *British Journal of Psychiatry* 180: 8–12.

# Environments of care

## Learning objectives

- Identify the current changes to service delivery in health care.
- Understand why current changes to service delivery in health care are necessary.
- Understand the role of primary, secondary and tertiary care (in national and private health services) in the provision of health care.
- Understand the role of patients and users in the development of health care services and why this is important.
- Understand the implications of increased patient and user involvement in health care and the ways in which patients and users are being supported to manage their own health and to become experts.
- Understand what patient choice means for health care users and how this can affect care delivery.

## Introduction

This chapter will discuss the environments in which health care is delivered. This will include a discussion of the current situation and changes to healthcare delivery, primary, secondary and tertiary care and the role of each of these. Healthcare provision by the National

Health Service will provide the main focus, but there will also be a discussion of private health care. The chapter will also include the increasing involvement of patients in the management of their care and the need to include patient/user perspectives in the development of health care as well as specific programmes aimed to help patients to manage their own health, such as the expert patient programme. The chapter will also include the recent initiative of patient choice and the impact of this on health care and its delivery.

Changes to the way that health care is delivered have played an important part in the modernisation of health services in the UK in recent years. These changes have included a move away from traditional views of single, separate healthcare institutions to the management of patient's health care across various healthcare organisations and their services. These changes have taken place, at least in part, as a result of an ageing population and the, somewhat related, increase in chronic disease and the associated costs of care.

Since the publication of the initiative for these changes – *The Coming of Age: Improving Care Services for Older People* (Audit Commission, 1997) – which indicated that insufficient investment in preventive and rehabilitation services was not only an inefficient use of an expensive resource but was also detrimental to patients' health and well-being, further work has supported its findings and the need for change to healthcare delivery. The Beds Inquiry (Department of Health, 2000a), for example, showed that two-thirds of hospital beds are occupied by people aged 65 years or more. Further, the incidence of long-term conditions is increasing (Department of Health, 1999, 2000b; World Health Organisation, 2002). These affect 17.5 million people in Great Britain, account for 80% of general practitioner (GP) consultations, 60% of hospital bed days and, in the over 65s, are likely to more than double by 2030 (Department of Health, 2005a). In addition to these changes in the age and health of the population, there have been changes to what patients and service users expect from health care. Patients want to be more involved in making decisions and choosing their health care (British Medical Association, 2000).

## The need for changes to service delivery in health care

The financial and other demands that have taken place as a result of changes to the age and health of the population have necessitated a move away from models of care that focus on the clinical component of health care (diagnostics and physiological management), exclude the patient component (education, support and motivation) and view the patient as a recipient. This has been, in part, because of increasing financial pressures to find the most efficient ways of delivering the most effective health care.

# Environments of care

## *The National Health Service*

Since its creation in 1948, the NHS has been providing care to patients throughout the UK. Today, people are treated faster and more effectively than ever before (NHS Confederation, 2006). This is despite the number of hospital beds having fallen by one-third in the past 20 years. When talking about the provision of health care and the NHS, most people immediately think of their local hospital. Changes to both the expectations of patients and to the health and age of the population in the UK have resulted in changes to the needs of the population and therefore the need for changes in the emphasis of health services (Department of Health, 2000a). At the same time as the number of beds has fallen, hospitals have seen a 57% increase in inpatients in the 20 years between 1984 and 2004, and a 341% increase in day cases (Department of Health, 2005b). These changes have occurred as a result of the following (NHS Confederation, 2006):

- Patients prefer to be treated somewhere other than an acute hospital.
- Care can be more effectively provided outside of the NHS.
- Technology has changed the type of treatment provided.
- Improvements to the management of chronic diseases.
- Reductions in first-time admissions to hospital as a result of changes to emergency care.
- The provision of specialist services rather than generic.
- Reductions in waiting times.

These changes have resulted in changes to the way in which health care is delivered and, in particular, to an increased emphasis on primary care in the provision of health care. Primary care covers a range of health and social care services between acute hospitals and a patient's home. While these (community) services have existed within the health service for a long time, recent changes to the way in which care is delivered has seen the development of primary care as a means of reducing unnecessary admissions to acute care and of ensuring timely and appropriate hospital discharge.

Where more specialised health care is required, patients are referred to secondary care – an acute hospital – to see a specialist/consultant. These hospitals have more elaborate diagnostic and treatment aids, which allow detailed examination of patients and the initiation of specialised treatments as necessary. In cases where such services are not sufficient, tertiary care, provided only at larger hospitals by consultants with special expertise, is sought. Tertiary care centres have the equipment and facilities required for handling complex cases.

While people are likely to receive the majority of their continuing care in primary care, it is recognised that most will require access to some areas of care offered elsewhere. For example, a person with diabetes may receive the majority of his/her care within primary care but may be referred to secondary or tertiary care for specific reasons, and then return to primary care. The provision of effective care therefore relies on the integration of skills from primary, secondary and tertiary care to achieve appropriate standards of care.

The traditional classification of primary, secondary and tertiary care (above) is based on the environment in which healthcare interventions take place, namely general practice or community care, district hospitals and regional centres. To some extent these terms also reflect a hierarchy of specialisation from general to more specialist services.

---

**Activity**

Think about some of the patients you see in the course of your work.

- Where (i.e. primary, secondary or tertiary care centres) do they receive the majority of their care?
- What contact, if any, do you have with these other centres?
- How does this affect the care that you are involved in?

---

## Private health care

The relationship between the public and private sectors in health care has been complicated since the start of the NHS in 1948. Reforms introduced in 1991 by the then Conservative Government sought to contain costs, maintain equity, improve efficiency and reduce waiting times. These created an 'internal market' in health care, in which publicly financed purchasers of care contracted for services with competing public and private providers. Until recently, the private sector has played a relatively minor role in the provision of health care in the UK compared to the role of the NHS. Early signs of an increase in private sector involvement included the privatisation of glasses, dentistry and longer-term care. The Labour Government's adoption of the Conservative's Private Finance Initiative (PFI), in which the private sector finance and build hospitals and the government contracts and pays to use these for 30 years, caused concern. Labour increased public, that is NHS, funding and aimed to increase capacity, efficiency, raise quality and reduce costs, by increasing competition and by using the private sector to operate on NHS patients.

Another increase in competitive pressure and change to the environment in which health care is delivered has occurred recently with the introduction of 'independent sector treatment centres' (ISTCs). These are built and staffed by private providers under government contracts: 'payment by results' (PBR), where these hospitals are paid a tariff for treating patients. Competitive pressures are further increased by the recent introduction of 'patient choice' in which patients needing hospital care can choose when, where and by whom they are treated.

---

**Activity**

- What do you think the main differences between private and NHS care are?
- Do you think it is good to have competition in health care?
- Why?

---

## User involvement in health care

As a result of recent and ongoing changes to the age and health of the population in the UK, and the associated costs of these changes, models of care that view the patient as participant are increasingly promoted (Department of Health, 1999, 2000a; World Health Organisation, 2002). Healthcare provision can be divided into a clinical component, which includes diagnostic interventions, monitoring and management of physiological indicators of the disease and pharmaceutical prescription, and a patient component, which includes patient education, social support and motivation. Traditional models of care that focus on the clinical component and exclude the patient component of care are no longer acceptable (Holman & Lorig, 2000; Wagner, 2001).

The evolving self-care agenda in the NHS is key to the development of a patient-centred health service and to the effective management of an ageing population and an increasing incidence of chronic disease (Department of Health, 2000a, 2005c). As part of this, the government has set a National Public Service Agreement target for improving outcomes for people with long-term conditions by reducing emergency bed days by 5% by 2008 (Department of Health, 2005a). This has been addressed, to some extent, by the move toward the increased use of primary care services in preference to secondary and tertiary care. To ensure that these aims are met, however, changes to the role of service users and patients in the management of their own health are also required. Patients with chronic disease(s) need to become experts in the management of their own care.

## *The expert patient and self-management*

Patient self-management: an 'individual's ability to manage symptoms, treatment, physical and psychosocial consequences and lifestyle changes inherent in living with a chronic condition' (Barlow, 2001, p. 546) is fundamental to user involvement in health care (Department of Health, 1999, 2000a; World Health Organisation, 2002). While they have recently been highlighted by healthcare reform, the concepts of patient self-management and of the patient as an expert are not new. Their origins are traceable through the Fabian welfare state's 'clean simplified living'; Beveridge's (1942) five giants of illness: 'want', 'idleness', 'ignorance', 'disease' and 'squalor'; and, more recently, in the 1970s to the Labour Government's focus on personal behaviour (Department of Health, 1976). More recently, the expert patient emerged in the White Paper *Saving Lives: Our Healthier Nation* (Department of Health, 1999), which developed the Green Paper 'on trying to get people to live healthy lives . . . by changing their lifestyle' (Department of Health, 1999, p. 2).

Defined as 'the individual's ability to manage symptoms, treatment, physical and psychosocial consequences and lifestyle changes inherent in living with a chronic condition' (Barlow, 2001, p. 546), self-management offers a way of bridging the gap between patients' needs and healthcare provision. Research findings from recent studies, primarily randomised controlled trials (RCT) based mainly in the USA, indicate that self-management increases self-efficacy, reduces GP visits (Barlow *et al.*, 2000), symptoms (Lorig *et al.*, 1999), costs (Liljas & Lahdensuo, 1997) and improves outcomes (Bodenheimer *et al.*, 2002).

## *The Expert Patients' Programme*

The Expert Patients' Programme (EPP) (Department of Health, 2001), is a self-management course that aims to develop the confidence and motivation of patients to use their own skills, information and professional services, to take effective control over life with a chronic condition. It was launched in the UK in 2001. In its current form, the EPP (Department of Health, 2001), is based on the Stanford Chronic Disease Self Management (CDSM) Programme model: a lay-led generic group programme for chronic disease conditions. The EPP delivers cognitive, generic information about relaxation, symptom management, exercise, nutrition, problem solving and communication to patients with chronic diseases. In essence it provides the patient component missing from many models of healthcare provision.

The EPP aims to increase capacity for self-care and self-management of chronic disease (Department of Health, 2001). The resultant outcomes should be (Department of Health, 2001):

- improved or stabilised symptoms, and reduced deterioration and complications;

- improved patient self-management of specific aspects of their condition, e.g. symptoms, medication;
- reduced incapacity caused by fatigue, low energy levels and emotional consequences;
- appropriate use of health and social care services and gaining/retaining employment;
- that patients are well informed, feel empowered and have higher self-esteem;
- that people with chronic disease contribute their skills and insights to improve services.

The programme comprises six, 2-hour long, weekly sessions delivered by lay leaders, most of whom have a long-term condition, and is based on developing the confidence and motivation of patients to use their skills, information and services to take effective control over their lives (NHS Expert Patients Programme, 2002). Cognitive, generic information about relaxation, symptom management, exercise, nutrition, problem solving and communication is delivered to groups of (a maximum of) 18 people. Since pilot EPPs were introduced in May 2002 over 1000 courses have been run by Primary Care Trusts (PCTs) and voluntary organisations, with an estimated total attendance of 13,000 (NHS, 2005), and plans exist to roll out the programme throughout the NHS by 2008 (Department of Health, 2004) (see http://www.expertpa tients.nhs.uk/ for further information).

---

**Activity**

In your nursing role, think about how patient self-management and the expert patient influences the way that you work:

- in relation to the way that care is delivered
- in relation to how patient involvement is promoted.

What do you think the advantages and disadvantages of patient self-management and the expert patient are?

- Advantages, e.g. involves patients in their own care.
- Disadvantages, e.g. some patients might not want to be involved.

---

# Patient choice

Patient choice forms a key element of the government's health policy. Initially triggered by the need to reduce waiting times, it is part of a wider set of policies designed to devolve NHS power, improve quality, and respond to the needs and expectations of patients and service users. Society is changing, not only in relation to age and health, but also in relation to lifestyles. People want more convenient health services that are tailored to their needs. In the national choice consultation (Department of Health, 2003), 76% of people said that the main health-care priority should be to involve people more in decisions about their illness and treatment. More recently, the British Social Attitudes Survey (Park, 2005) confirmed that 65% of people want to be able to choose their treatment, 63% their hospital and 53% the date and time of their appointment. New research carried out for the Department of Health by RAND Europe, the King's Fund and City University (Burge *et al.*, 2006) found that clinical quality would exert the largest influence if people were making a choice of hospital.

The NHS, private health care and social care systems now offer more choice and more control for patients and service users than ever before. Evaluation of the scheme has had largely positive results, with 67% of patients in the London patient choice project choosing to go to another hospital for faster treatment, and 97% of those patients saying that they would recommend the scheme (Picker Institute, 2005). Whenever possible, patients have an informed choice of treatment options, treatment providers, location for receiving care, type of ongoing care and choice at the end of life (Department of Health, 2006).

Patient choice of hospital is inextricably linked with the payment by results system being rolled out across the UK. Under payment by results (PBR), the money that hospitals receive is linked directly to the amount of work carried out by individual hospitals, with the majority of prices per patient fixed by a national tariff. In theory this provides a financial incentive for hospitals to attract patients through improved quality, and to boost 'surpluses' by reducing costs below the nationally fixed price. In practice, however, the move to PBR raises some concern about the quality of care and the possibility of hospitals 'cherry picking' less complicated cases. PBR only measures activity, and reflects the previous, somewhat biased, method for measuring productivity in health care (Office of National Statistics, 2006).

As part of patient choice, 'Choose and Book' is one of the first schemes that bring about this change, allowing patients to choose the hospital or other organisation where they will be seen by a specialist. Choose and Book is a new service that allows patients to choose a local or foundation trust hospital or clinic and to book an appointment with a specialist and to choose the date and time of their appointment. For patients, the key benefits include improved access to hospitals and real choice about when and where their hospital appointment will be. For clinicians and staff, tracking the progress of referrals is automated, with considerable potential saving in administrative time. It is anticipated that non-attendance at appointments will fall because of the choice provided. Since mid 2004, Choose and Book has been introduced across England and will eventually be available to all patients.

Since December 2005, all patients referred by their GP for a specialist consultation at a hospital outpatient department are offered a choice of at least four hospitals, both NHS and private. From 2008, the government promises to offer all patients the choice of any hospital, public or private, anywhere in the country. A recent MORI survey (2005) showed that three out of four people would be happy to go to either an NHS or a private provider for their treatment (see www.nhs.uk/choosean dbook for more information).

---

**Activity**

What do you think the advantages and disadvantages of patient choice are?

- Advantages, e.g. patients can decide where they will receive their care.
- Disadvantages, e.g. some patients will have to choose the hospital closest to them because care elsewhere will mean travel for them and for their family, so it does not mean they have real choice.

---

**Summary**

- Health care can be delivered in primary, secondary and tertiary care settings, both within and outside the NHS.
- The need for increased efficiency in healthcare delivery has meant that there is now competition for the provision of health care.
- The increasing involvement of patients in their own health care has resulted in changes to the way care is delivered.
- Patients have more choice than ever before about when, where and from whom they will receive health care.
- Patients are encouraged to take a more active role in their health care and can attend programmes to enable them to do so.

# References

Audit Commission (1997) *The Coming of Age: Improving Care Services for Older People.* Audit Commission, London.

Barlow, J H (2001) How to use education as an intervention in osteoarthritis. *Best Practice and Research in Clinical Rheumatology* 15 (4): 545–58.

Barlow, J H, Turner, A P & Wright, C C (2000) A randomised controlled study of an arthritis self-management programme in the UK. *Health Education Research: Theory and Practice* 15 (6): 665–80.

Bodenheimer, T, Wagner, E H & Grumbach, K (2002) Improving primary care for patients with chronic illness. *Journal of American Medical Association* 288 (14): 1775–9.

British Medical Association (2000) What sort of healthcare does the public expect, want or need? *Healthcare Funding Review Research Report Summary.* BMA, London. Available at www.bma.org.uk/ap.nsf/Content/Healthcare+funding+review+research+report+1

Burge, P, Devlin, N, Appleby, J, Gallo, F, Nason, E & Ling, T (eds) (2006) *Understanding Patients' Choices at the Point of Referral.* A report for the Department of Health. RAND Publ., Cambridge.

Department of Health (1976) *Prevention and Health, Everybody's Business: A Reassessment of Public and Personal Health.* HMSO, London.

Department of Health (1999) *Saving Lives: Our Healthier Nation.* HMSO, London.

Department of Health (2000a) *Shaping the Future NHS: Long Term Planning for Hospitals and Related Services.* HMSO, London.

Department of Health (2000b) *The NHS Plan: A Plan for Investment, a Plan for Reform.* HMSO, London.

Department of Health (2001) *The Expert Patient A New Approach to Chronic Disease Management for the 21st Century.* HMSO, London.

Department of Health (2003) *Choice, Responsiveness and Equity National Consultation.* HMSO, London.

Department of Health (2004) *The NHS Improvement Plan: Putting People at the Heart of Public Services.* HMSO, London.

Department of Health (2005a) *Supporting People with Long Term Conditions. An NHS and Social Care Model to Support Local Innovation and Integration.* HMSO, London.

Department of Health (2005b) *Bed Availability and Occupancy.* HMSO, London.

Department of Health (2005c). *Self-Care – A Real Choice. Self Care Support – A Practical Option.* HMSO, London.

Department of Health (2006) *Choice Matters: Increasing Choice Improves Patients' Experiences. Choose and Book.* HMSO, London.

Holman, H & Lorig, K (2000) Patients as partners in managing chronic disease. *British Medical Journal* 320 (7234): 526–7.

Liljas, B & Lahdensuo A (1997) Is asthma self-management cost-effective? *Patient Education and Counseling* 32 (1 Supp.): S97–104.

Lorig, K R, Sobel, D S, Stewart, A L, Brown, B W Jr, Bandura, A, Ritter, P, Gonzalez, V M, Laurent, D D & Holman H R (1999) Evidence suggesting that a chronic disease self-management programme can improve health status while reducing hospitalisation. A randomised controlled trial. *Medical Care* 37 (1): 5–14.

MORI (2005) *What will people choose when choice goes live.* MORI/24267 poll for the Department of Health. Available at http://www.dh.gov.uk/asset Root/04/12/58/28/04125828.pdf

NHS (2005) *About Expert Patients: EPP Progress.* Available at http://www. expertpatients.nhs.uk/about_progress.shtml

NHS Confederation (2006) *Shaping The Health Debate: Why We Need Fewer Hospital Beds.* The NHS Confederation, London.

NHS Expert Patients Programme (2002) *Self-management for Long Term Health Conditions: A Handbook for People with Chronic Health Conditions.* Bull Publ. Co., Boulder Colorado.

Office of National Statistics (2006) *Public Service productivity.* Available at http://www.statistics.gov.uk/articles/nojournal/PublicServiceProductivi tyHealth(27_2_06).pdf

Park, A (ed.) (2005) *British Social Attitudes Survey 22nd Report.* National Centre for Social Research, London.

Picker Institute (2005) *London Patient Choice Project. Patients' Experience of Choosing Where to Undergo Surgical Treatment.* Picker Institute, London.

Wagner, E H (2001) Meeting the needs of chronically ill people. *British Medical Journal* 323 (7319): 845–946.

World Health Organisation (2002) *Innovative Care for Chronic Conditions: Building Blocks for Action.* WHO, Geneva, Switzerland.

Section 4

# Principles of Professional Issues

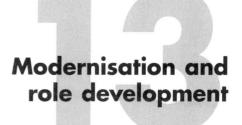

# Modernisation and role development

## Introduction

In this chapter the modernisation of the NHS will be outlined. The development of both new roles for nurses and the clinical skills required to fulfil these new roles will be discussed.

## Modernisation

The past decade has witnessed great changes in the way health care is delivered in the UK. The UK government's plan for modernisation and reform in the NHS dates back to 1997, and the years following have seen a number of key White Papers produced consecutively by the Department of Health. A summary of these key Department of Health papers is presented below.

## The new NHS: modern, dependable (1997)

This paper set out the government's plans for modernisation of the NHS. The Prime Minister declared that this paper marked a turning point for the NHS by replacing the internal market with integrated care, putting money into frontline patient care, ensuring high-quality care and introducing national standards of care. The approach aimed to combine efficiency and quality with a belief in fairness and partnership. The intention of this White Paper was to begin a process of modernisation, within the NHS, to provide more efficient and effective services to the public.

## A first class service: quality in the new NHS (1998)

*A First Class Service* outlined how fair access and high-quality care would be achieved across the NHS. It declared that unacceptable variations in standards of care must come to an end and presented the changes that were to take place in order to achieve this goal: 'The objective is to ensure fair access to effective, prompt high quality care wherever a patient is treated across the NHS' (Department of Health, 1998, p. 6).

*A First Class Service* laid down a plan for setting, delivering and monitoring national standards. Both National Service Frameworks and the National Institute for Health and Clinical Excellence set clear national standards of service (discussed in further detail in Chapter 14). The system for local delivery of these standards included a new system of clinical governance, a process of lifelong learning and professional self-regulation. Three new mechanisms were set up to oversee the monitoring of these standards:

- The Commission for Health Improvement, this was superseded in April 2005 by the Healthcare Commission (see later in this chapter for more information).
- A national framework for assessing performance, which included the introduction of NHS performance indicators (NHS Executive, 1999a). The intention was to provide useful information about the quality, efficiency and outcomes of NHS services (NHS Executive, 2000).
- The National Patient and User Survey. This led to the first national survey of NHS patients and aimed at ensuring that patients had a voice.

## Making a difference: strengthening the nursing, midwifery and health visiting contribution to health and healthcare (1999)

This paper was perhaps the most important of the White Papers in relation to the role of nursing in modernisation. It recognised that nurses, midwives and health visitors are vital to the NHS and crucial to the government's plans for the modernisation of services. It recognised the constraints on nursing development and innovation in the current structures, and aimed to look at ways of strengthening the nursing, midwifery and health visiting contribution to health care and relating these to the changing needs of the patient.

The paper set out the strategic intentions for modern nursing. These included a drive to recruit more nurses through:

- a major expansion in workforce
- additional training places
- a campaign to attract people into nursing and workforce planning for future staffing requirements.

Education and training were to be strengthened through:

- more career opportunities
- higher quality placements
- teacher support and practical skills training
- improvement in leadership in nurse education
- a framework for post-registration education
- continuing professional development.

Other key aspects included:

- developing a modern career framework
- improving working lives
- nurse roles in enhancing the quality of care
- strengthening nurse leadership
- modernising professional regulation
- working in new ways.

## The NHS plan: a plan for investment, a plan for reform (2000)

The Department of Health asserted that the NHS Plan constituted the biggest change to healthcare in England since the NHS was formed in 1948. It outlined a new delivery system for the NHS and set out how increased funding and reform aimed to redress geographical inequalities, improve service standards and extend patient choice. The NHS Plan was produced following a major public consultation, which highlighted that the public wanted more and better paid staff, reduced waiting times, high-quality patient-centred care and improvements in local hospitals and surgeries.

Crucially, it identified that there was a lack of national standards and that staff were working in old-fashioned ways. The plan aimed to address this by investment and reform, in which staff had the opportunity to expand their roles and patients were given new powers. The overall aim was to improve care for patients, for example by setting targets for shorter waiting times.

The implementation of the NHS Plan (Department of Health, 2000) was, perhaps, one of the biggest stepping-stones in advancing nursing practice. It challenges what can be described as professional boundaries. These boundaries restrict the roles that staff were permitted to fulfil, based on their professional identity, rather than on the basis of their knowledge or competence (Taylor–Hewitt, 2003).

The NHS Plan (Department of Health, 2000) stated that, for the first time, nurses and other staff, not just in some places but everywhere, will have greater opportunity to extend their roles. The objective was to liberate the talent and skills of all the workforce so that every patient gets the right care in the right place at the right time. It was in the NHS Plan that the Chief Nursing Officer identified ten key roles for nurses, which identified new and expanded roles for nurses, to quantify their contribution to the new NHS.

The government has introduced several initiatives aimed at redefining the traditional structure of the NHS, some of which have already been mentioned above. Since the publication of the NHS Plan numerous Department of Health documents have been produced to support the implementation of the principles outlined in 'The plan'. More information on these can be found on the Department of Health website (http://www.dh.gov.uk).

---

**Activity**

Visit the Department of Health website:

- What other White Papers and documents have been produced since the NHS Plan?
- Which are of most importance to nursing?
- Choose one document and summarise the implications for nursing practice.

---

# New initiatives

A number of new services have been introduced to assist in the implementation of these changes. Examples of these include the following.

## The NHS modernisation agency

The Modernisation Agency was established in April 2001 to support the NHS and its partner organisations in England, in the task of modernising services and improving experiences and outcomes for patients. It was superseded on 1 July 2005 by the **NHS Institute for Innovation** and **Improvement.** The Institute was an indication of improvement and change for the NHS in England. Established as a Special Health Authority in England, and based on the campus of the University of Warwick, the mission of the NHS Institute was to support the NHS and its workforce in the move towards the delivery of world-class health and healthcare for patients and public. It aimed to achieve this by encouraging innovation and developing capability at the frontline (more information can be found at http://www.institute. nhs.uk/).

## NHS direct

NHS direct was established in 1998 with the remit to provide easier and faster health advice and information to the public. The service has developed and is now open 24 hours a day 7 days a week, all year round. It now has national telephone coverage; which was achieved in November 2000. NHS Direct is, in fact, the world's largest provider of telephone healthcare advice (National Audit Office, 2002). The full-time equivalent of 1150 qualified nurses in 22 call-receiving sites provide advice to callers using advanced computer clinical decision support software. In addition, the online service provides an e-mail health information enquiry service and web links to health information.

The government claims that NHS Direct facilitates better access to NHS services and improvements in out-of-hours services (National Audit Office, 2002), declaring that it is at the forefront of modernising the NHS. The National Audit Office (2002) reported that the implementation of NHS Direct, so far, had been a success and made recommendations on how to build on that success (more information can be found at http://www.nhsdirect.nhs.uk/).

## The healthcare commission

The Healthcare Commission is an independent body set up to promote and drive improvement in the quality of healthcare and public health. In the NHS Plan (Department of Health, 2000) the government originally sanctioned the setting up of the **Commission for Health Improvement** (CHI). The Healthcare Commission replaced the CHI in April 2005; it also took over responsibilities from the private and voluntary healthcare functions of the National Care Standards Commission and covers the elements of the Audit Commission's work that relate to efficiency, effectiveness and economy of health care.

The function of the Healthcare Commission is to inspect the quality and value for money of health care and public health, equip patients and the public with the best possible information about the provision of health care, and promote improvements in health care and public health. The commission website outlines its statutory duties in England. These are presented in Box 13.1.

---

**Box 13.1 The Healthcare Commission: statutory duties.**

- Assess the management, provision and quality of NHS health care and public health services
- Review the performance of each NHS trust and award an annual performance rating
- Regulate the independent healthcare sector through registration, annual inspection, monitoring complaints and enforcement
- Publish information about the state of health care
- Consider complaints about NHS organisations that the organisations themselves have not resolved
- Promote the coordination of reviews and assessments carried out by ourselves and others
- Carry out investigations of serious failures in the provision of health care

---

The Healthcare Commission is required to pay particular attention to:

- the availability of, access to, quality and effectiveness of health care
- the economy and efficiency of the provision of health care
- the availability and quality of information provided to the public about health care
- the need to safeguard and promote the rights and welfare of children and the effectiveness of measures taken to do so.

More information can be found at http://www.healthcarecommission. org.uk

---

**Activity**

Think about the area in which you practice.

- What role does the Healthcare Commission play in relation to your practice?

Find out if there has been a Healthcare Commission visit to your organisation. If a report is available (usually in the library), summarise the main findings and find out whether the recommendations have been put into practice.

---

## *Role development*

The roles of all healthcare workers in the UK have been affected by the government's national initiatives for modernising health care, and the role of the nurse, in particular, has changed considerably over the past decade. In line with government reform, nursing has been responsive to the changing needs of health care. The government agenda has placed particular emphasis on the expanding role of the nurse in increasing the efficiency and quality of service provision within the NHS. The Scope of Professional Practice (UKCC, 1992) has enabled the development of new nursing roles (Walsh *et al.*, 1999). Over a decade ago, the Scope of Professional Practice relaxed the restraints that had constrained nursing practice, allowing nurses greater freedom to expand their roles to benefit patient care. This document emphasised knowledge, judgement, accountability and skill, and helped nurses to make a cultural shift, from delegated tasks to greater professional autonomy (Walsgrove & Fulbrook, 2005).

Some questions have arisen about why advanced nursing roles have evolved, and concerns have been expressed in relation to the effect this may have on traditional roles of nurses when nurses are undertaking tasks previously carried out by junior doctors. However, the notion of extending nursing roles has been sustained largely due to the clear indications that in doing this, patient care can be improved (Dolan *et al.*, 1997; DeCarlo, 2005).

As a result of the NHS Plan, nurses and midwives were empowered to undertake a wider range of clinical activity. The government's strategy for nursing and midwifery, as highlighted in *The NHS Plan* (Department of Health, 2000) and *Making a Difference* (Department of Health, 1999), recognised the need to introduce new roles and new ways of working for nurses and midwives to help improve services and drive up the quality of patient treatment and care. The Chief Nursing Officer at the time identified ten key roles for nurses (Box 13.2); these have formed the core of the development of roles and nurses' contribution to the new NHS (Department of Health, 2000).

# New roles and new skills for nurses

One result of the flurry of activity around the modernisation of the NHS is the development of nursing as a profession in previously unprecedented ways. Nurses are undertaking new roles and new skills that were not previously thought possible. The balance between advancing nursing and ensuring that the fundamentals of care are delivered has led to both the introduction and re-introduction of a number of roles for nurses. In the UK, these include the nurse consultant, the matron, the nurse practitioner and the emergency care practitioner.

---

> **Box 13.2 Chief Nursing Officer's ten key roles for nurses (Department of Health, 2000).**
>
> (1) To order diagnostic investigations such as pathology tests and X-rays
> (2) To make and receive referrals direct, say, to a therapist or pain consultant
> (3) To admit and discharge patients for specified conditions and within agreed protocols
> (4) To manage patient caseloads, say for diabetes or rheumatology
> (5) To run clinics, say, for ophthalmology or dermatology
> (6) To prescribe medicines and treatments
> (7) To carry out a wide range of resuscitation procedures, including defibrillation
> (8) To perform minor surgery and outpatient procedures
> (9) To triage patients using the latest IT to the most appropriate health professional
> (10) To take a lead in the way local health services are organised and in the way that they are run

With other roles, including healthcare assistant and nurse specialists, expanding and extending to incorporate new ways of working.

## Nurse consultants

The introduction of the nurse consultant role was a direct response to an announcement made by the British Prime Minister in 1998, who stated that he wanted to see nurse consultant posts established in the NHS. This was followed by plans for the introduction being outlined in *Making a Difference: Strengthening the Nursing, Midwifery and Health Visiting Contribution to Health and Healthcare* (Department of Health, 1999). NHS trusts were then invited to submit to Regional Offices proposals to establish such posts, and eventually the first nurse consultant appointments were made in 2000.

Specific guidance for the introduction included information on how the role should be structured. Nurse consultants, irrespective of the field in which they practised or the service in which they were based, had their posts structured around four core functions of the role:

- an expert practice function;
- a professional leadership and consultancy function;
- an education, training and development function; and
- a practice and service development, research and evaluation function.

These four core functions are explained in detail in Health Service Circular 1999/217, Sections 7–15 (NHS Executive, 1999b). They are summarised in Table 13.1.

**Purpose**

The purpose of the nurse consultant role is to:

> *Help to provide better outcomes for patients by improving services and quality, to strengthen leadership and to provide a new career opportunity to help retain experienced and expert nurse, midwives and health visitors in practice* (NHS Executive, 1999).

It was expected that the introduction of the role would lead to an improvement in both the quality of patient care and also to the development of better services for patients, which ultimately would lead to better outcomes for patients. Secondly, the intention was to provide nurses with new a promotion route to enable experienced nurses to remain clinical, working with patients, as opposed to moving into management, research or education, which were previously the only promotion routes in nursing. The implementation of the role has been the subject of much debate and discussion, and the success of the role has been varied (Guest *et al.*, 2004; Woodward *et al.*, 2005).

## *The matron*

The (modern) matron role was introduced into the National Health Service (NHS) in 2001 as part of the NHS Plan (Department of Health, 2000), which set out the government's strategy for modernising all aspects of the NHS, improving the quality of care, and making the service more responsive to the needs of patients and their families. A public consultation, which preceded the NHS Plan (Department of Health, 2000), found that both patients and their relatives were often concerned about a lack of consistent responsibility for care, and the lack of authority of nurses to address shortcomings that were fundamental to patient care. The consultation recognised that there was a perceived need for a strong clinical leader with clear authority at ward and department level. In response, the NHS Plan identified the need for: 'A new generation of managerial and clinical leaders, including modern matrons, who would have the authority to get the basics right on the ward' (Department of Health, 2000, p. 23).

It proposed that every hospital should appoint 'modern matrons' in order to secure the highest standards of clinical care by providing leadership to professional and direct-care staff, and to provide a visible, accessible and authoritative presence in care settings – someone to whom patients and families could turn for assistance, advice and support. The Health Service Circular Guidance Document 2001/010 (Department of Health, 2001, p. 2) described the matron as: 'A strong

**Table 13.1** Four core functions of the nurse consultant (NHS Executive, 1999b).

| Core function | Description |
|---|---|
| The expert practice function | Nurse, midwife and health visitor consultants will be senior, experienced practitioners who are experts in their field. The main element of all posts will be the provision of expert nursing, midwifery or health visiting. At least half the time available should be spent working in practice with patients, clients or communities. Nurse consultants are expected to exercise a high degree of personal and professional autonomy and make critical judgments to satisfy the expectations and demands of the job. They will be expected to draw on advanced knowledge and exercise professional skills of the highest order |
| The professional leadership and consultancy function | Nurse consultants will be senior practice-based roles comprising a significant professional leadership function. Nurse consultants will be supported in exercising leadership to support and inspire colleagues, to improve standards and quality and to develop professional practice. Setting standards, developing and promoting best practice is a key part of the role and demands leadership and change management skills. They will have a crucial role in clinical governance, providing expert input and working to secure quality improvement, including influencing other disciplines to help deliver better services |
| The education, training and development function | Nurse consultants will be expected to contribute to the education, training and development of nurses, midwives, health visitors and others. They will help to identify and respond to learning needs at individual, team and organisational levels. They will focus on experienced colleagues who need to develop advanced knowledge and skills. Their practice expertise will enable them to play a key role in helping to integrate theory and practice and sustain productive partnerships with universities. Many nurse consultant posts will be established with formal university links to support and advance these goals. |
| The practice and service development, research and evaluation function | Nurse consultant posts will help develop professional practice locally (and nationally through professional associations). They are likely to include key responsibilities associated with the promotion of evidence-based practice, with setting, monitoring and auditing standards, and with the identification and promotion of measures to secure and evaluate quality improvement. They will have a track record of scholarship and the appraisal and application of research in practice, and in many cases formal research expertise |

clinical leader with clear authority at ward level who is highly visible, accessible and easily identifiable by patients and has real authority to ensure that the basics of care are correct'.

While accountable for a group of wards/departments, the three key elements central to the role of the matrons are (Department of Health, 2001):

(1) Providing a visible, accessible and authoritative presence in ward/ department settings to whom patients and their families can turn for assistance, advice and support.
(2) Securing and assuring the highest standards of clinical care by providing leadership to the professional and direct-care staff within the group of wards/departments for which they are accountable.
(3) Ensuring that administrative and support services are designed and delivered to achieve the highest standards of care within the group of wards/departments for which they are accountable.

In April 2002, the Department of Health published *Modern Matrons in the NHS: A Progress Report* (Department of Health, 2002a). Just one year after plans to introduce the role there were 1900 matrons in post, nearly four times as many as anticipated. The report highlighted some examples of good practice that matrons were involved in, which included: monitoring cleanliness, preventing hospital-acquired infection, empowering nurses and resolving problems for patients and their relatives. The report also described how some matrons were successfully using the *Essence of Care* toolkit to raise standards of nursing. It also stated that matrons would be expected to provide annual reports about local progress in implementing the Chief Nursing Officer's ten key roles for nurses (Department of Health, 2002b).

In addition to the 2002 report, the Department of Health has issued further details outlining the roles and responsibilities of the matron role: 'Matrons have the power to re-design NHS care at the front line to make it patient centred. They have sufficient authority and support to get things done and make change happen' (Department of Health, 2003).

In *Modern Matrons – Improving the Patient Experience* (Department of Health, 2003), the Chief Nursing Officer commented that the range of functions that matrons perform, and the ways they could improve the patient experience, was 'even greater than originally foreseen'. The report set out more examples of good practice, and highlighted what were now defined as the 'ten key responsibilities' of modern matrons (Box 13.3).

The matron role provides NHS Trusts with the opportunity to strengthen nursing leadership and impact on care delivery in ways that

---

> **Box 13.3 Ten key responsibilities of modern matrons (Department of Health, 2003).**
>
> (1) Leading by example
> (2) Making sure patients get quality care
> (3) Ensuring staffing is appropriate to patient needs
> (4) Empowering nurses to take on a wider range of clinical tasks
> (5) Improving hospital cleanliness
> (6) Ensuring patients' nutritional needs are met
> (7) Improving wards for patients
> (8) Making sure patients are treated with respect
> (9) Preventing hospital-acquired infection
> (10) Resolving problems for patients and their relatives by building closer relationships

address the fundamental needs of patients and their families. It is, however, a complex role and one whose effectiveness will be determined, at least to some extent, by the context in which matrons work, on the limits of their authority, their resources, the nature of their working relationships and the extent to which their role is seen as central to care provision (Read *et al.*, 2005).

## Nurse practitioners

New ways of working and the need to ensure that care is delivered to the right patient, in the right place at the right time have led to the development and increase in the number of nurse practitioner roles in primary and secondary care settings. Nursing is at the forefront of delivering high-quality care for patients. *The Scope of Professional Practice* (UKCC, 1992) paved the way for nurses to progress and adapt to include extended roles within their jobs. This expansion and extension of roles by nurses also led to the development of nurse practitioner roles.

Walsh *et al.* (1999) argue that only nurses who have advanced their knowledge and skills through education and experience can exercise increasing clinical discretion and accept greater responsibility through advanced practice, and thus be considered to be nurse practitioners. Nurse practitioners have increased their knowledge and skills to enable them to undertake the whole-patient assessment and be able to order appropriate tests. Although it is argued that nurse practitioners are expensive to train, there is evidence to suggest that the role is effective (Smith & Hall, 2003).

**Activity**

Do you have any experience of working with nurse consultants, matrons or nurse practitioners?

- What was it like to work with people in each of the different roles?
- How do their roles differ?
- How are their roles similar?
- How have you developed your own role?

The development of a range of clinical skills and competencies for nurse practitioners ensures a more timely and appropriate response to patients' needs. It equips nurse practitioners with the necessary skills and knowledge to assess and examine patients. The ultimate aim is to improve the quality and provision of patient care.

# Regulation

Along with new nursing roles obviously comes the extension of nursing practice, and nurses must be explicitly aware of their roles and responsibilities, both professionally and legally. Currently no UK-wide standards exist for this level of practice. Nurses with the same job title are, in fact, doing many different things. This is confusing within the profession, to other professionals and, more importantly, to the public. The Nursing and Midwifery Council (NMC) currently registers all nurses, midwives and specialty community public health nurses, as well as setting standards for education, training and conduct. The NMC proposes to establish a framework for a standard for a level of nursing practice beyond initial registration, i.e. advanced practice, and to set a standard that the public can expect of any nurse who is working at this level (more information about this can be found in Chapter 16).

**Summary**

- A number of key White Papers have been produced by the Department of Health to outline the way that health care in the UK is to be modernised.
- The modernisation of the NHS has led to great changes to the way in which all healthcare staff work and deliver care.
- A number of new services have been set up to help deliver this agenda.
- The expansion and extension of nurses' roles has led to the development of a new range of skills and roles for nurses.

# References

DeCarlo, L (2005) Advanced practice nurse entrepreneurs in a multidisciplinary surgical assisting partnership. *Association of Operating Room Nurses Journal* 82 (3): 418–30.

Department of Health (1997) *The New NHS; Modern, Dependable.* The Stationery Office, London.

Department of Health (1998) *A First Class Service: Quality in the New NHS.* The Stationery Office, London.

Department of Health (1999) *Making a Difference: Strengthening the Nursing Midwifery and Health Visiting Contribution to Health and Healthcare.* The Stationery Office, London.

Department of Health (2000) *The NHS Plan: A Plan for Investment. A Plan for Reform.* The Stationery Office, London.

Department of Health (2001) *Implementing The NHS Plan – Modern Matrons.* Health Service Circular 2001/010. The Stationery Office, London.

Department of Health (2002a) *Modern Matrons in the NHS: A Progress Report.* HMSO, London.

Department of Health (2002b) *Implementing The NHS Plan – 10 Key Roles for Nurses.* HMSO, London.

Department of Health (2003) *Modern Matrons – Improving the Patient Experience.* HMSO, London.

Dolan, B, Dale, J & Morley, V (1997) Nurse practitioners: the role in A and E and primary care. *Nursing Standard* 11 (17): 33–7.

Guest, D, Peccei, R, Rosenthal, P, Redfern, J, Wilson-Barnett, J, Dewe, P, Coster, S, Evans, A & Sundbury, A (2004) *An evaluation of the impact of nurse, midwife and health visitor consultants.* Unpublished report, King's College, London.

NHS Executive (1999a) *Improving Quality and Performance in the New NHS: Clinical Indicators and High Level Performance Indicators.* Health Service Circular 1999/139. NHS Executive, Leeds.

NHS Executive (1999b) *Nurse, Midwife and Health Visitor Consultants; Establishing Posts and Making Appointments.* Health Service Circular 1999/217. NHS Executive, Leeds.

NHS Executive (2000) *Improving quality and performance in the New NHS: NHS Performance Indicators.* Health Service Circular 2000/023. NHS Executive, Leeds.

National Audit Office (2002) *NHS Direct in England: Report by the Comptroller and Auditor General.* HC 505. The Stationery Office, London.

Read, S, Ashman, M, Scott, C & Savage, J (2005) *Evaluation of the Modern Matron Role in a Sample of NHS Trusts. Executive Summary.* University of Sheffield, Royal College of Nursing, London.

Smith, S L & Hall, M A (2003) Developing a neonatal workforce: role evolution and retention of advanced neonatal nurse practitioners. *Archives of Disease in Childhood Fetal And Neonatal Edition* 88: 426.

Taylor-Hewitt, J (2003) Nurses' role in the New NHS: standardisation of practice. *British Journal of Nursing* 12 (7): 436–43.

UKCC (United Kingdom Central Council for Nursing, Midwifery and Health Visiting) (1992) *The Scope of Professional Practice.* UKCC, London.

Walsgrove, H & Fulbrook, P (2005) Advancing the clinical perspective: a practice development project to develop the nurse practitioner role in an acute hospital trust. *Journal of Clinical Nursing* 14: 444–55.

Walsh, M, Crumbie, A & Reveley, S (1999) *Nurse Practitioners – Clinical Skills and Professional Issues.* Butterworth Heineman, Oxford.

Woodward, V A, Webb, C & Prowse M (2005) Nurse consultants: their characteristics and achievements. *Journal of Clinical Nursing* 14: 845–54.

# Frameworks for best practice

14

## Learning objectives

- Understand the principles of clinical governance and how it applies to healthcare delivery.
- Understand the models of clinical governance and how they are used by healthcare organisations.
- Identify factors to be considered in the implementation of clinical governance.
- Identify and understand the role of supporting mechanisms for the implementation of clinical governance.
- Identify sources of patient support when things go wrong.
- Understand the importance of setting, implementing and monitoring targets in health care.
- Demonstrate the importance of clinical audit and benchmarking to establish and maintain high standards of care.

## Introduction

In this chapter the frameworks that ensure the effective delivery of health care will be discussed. This includes a brief discussion of how and why clinical governance developed; models of clinical governance and how they are used in healthcare organisations; the implementation of clinical governance, including patient and organisational support mechanisms; and the cyclical nature of clinical governance and ways to evaluate it.

## Clinical governance

The term 'clinical governance' first appeared in UK health policy documents following the election of the Labour Government in 1997 (Department of Health, 1997). Since then, it has been the driving force for quality improvement in UK health care. Clinical governance emerged as a result of the need to improve the quality and consistency of care across the NHS. *An Organisation with a Memory* (Department of Health, 2000a) recognised that mistakes are made and it is important to learn from these mistakes. It also highlighted the need for a national system to help protect patients from these mistakes. The clinical governance framework provides a way in which the NHS can deal with, and learn from, adverse healthcare events. Its introduction was an important way forward in health care, as this was the first time that a national system for reporting such events had been introduced. This was reinforced by it becoming a legal obligation, as outlined in *The Health Act* (Department of Health, 1999a). Under this Act, chief executives of NHS healthcare organisations are held accountable for ensuring that clinical governance arrangements are in place, are supported within their organisation and make a real difference to patient care. While the papers published in the area (Department of Health, 1998, 1999b; Scally & Donaldson, 1998) do not use a standard definition of clinical governance, they include a number of common areas. Effective clinical governance should ensure (Commission for Health Improvement, 2002):

* continuous improvement of patient services and care
* a patient-centred approach that includes treating patients courteously, involving them in decisions about their care and keeping them informed
* a commitment to quality, which ensures that health professionals are up to date in their practice and properly supervised where necessary
* a reduction of the risk from clinical errors and adverse events as well as a commitment to learn from mistakes and share that learning with others.

*Clinical governance can be defined as a framework through which NHS organisations are accountable for continuously improving the quality of their services and safeguarding high standards of care by creating an environment in which excellence in clinical care will flourish* (Department of Health, 1998, p. 33).

Clinical governance is the framework through which nurses, as part of health care organisations, can ensure that healthcare delivery is safe, of a consistently high quality, patient-centred and constantly improving. This is carried out through a process that involves setting, implementing and monitoring targets for standards of quality, and by making sure that the most appropriate systems, structures and culture are in place.

Several factors can be used to determine if clinical governance is effective in an organisation. These include (Scally & Donaldson, 1998):

- clear lines of responsibility and accountability for the quality of care
- patient satisfaction
- effective information management systems
- a comprehensive programme of quality improvement systems, including clinical audit, evidence-based practice and clinical guidelines
- clear risk-management policies
- established education and training plans
- procedures for all professional groups to identify and remedy poor performance.

---

**Activity**

Think about the clinical governance arrangements in your place of work.

- What do you know about them?

Think about this in relation to the list above, which includes factors that can be used to determine if clinical governance is effective.

- What systems do you know of that are in place to gauge patient satisfaction?
- Are you aware of any clinical audits being carried out in your area?
- How is poor performance managed?

---

# Models of clinical governance

There are several models for defining and implementing clinical governance.

## The temple model

The temple model aims to make the patient an equal partner in his or her own health care (Hallet & Thompson, 2000). One of the ways to do this is by providing patients with information and seeking their view-points about the service they receive. Nurses have a key role to play in offering advice and information to patients, in seeking feedback and improving the quality of health care. Patient participation (discussed further in Chapter 6) is crucial to clinical governance, both at the organisational and individual patient level. To bring about quality improvement in health care, it is vital that the highest level of participation from patients and carers is encouraged and achieved whenever possible.

In the temple model, systems awareness, teamwork, communication, ownership and leadership help integrate the more technical tools of clinical governance and create the right culture to achieve beneficial change (Hallet & Thompson, 2000):

- Systems awareness: how (not by whom) things are done.
- Teamwork: ensuring teams work together in harmony.
- Communication: making sure everyone, including the patient, knows what is happening and why. Listening is as important as talking.
- Ownership: ensuring everyone has ownership in quality improvement and have a part to play.
- Leadership: effective leadership of both clinical and general management teams and activities is important if the organisation is to stay focused.

The temple model also recognises the more technical, or process, elements needed to implement clinical governance. These are (Hallet & Thompson, 2000):

- Ensuring that clinical effectiveness is high.
- Making sure that good risk-management processes are in place.
- The patient experience: seeking the views of the patient is central.
- Communication effectiveness: there needs to be a recognition, for instance, that communication is a two-way process. Communication needs to be more than top down.
- Resource effectiveness: is the best use being made of all available resources?
- Strategic effectiveness: making sure that clinical governance is written into all organisational planning, for example.
- Learning effectiveness: making sure that lessons really are being learnt and acted upon.

Figure 14.1 illustrates the seven 'pillars' that provide the support for the patient–professional partnership, which is at the heart of clinical governance and the temple model.

### The Commission for Health Improvement model of clinical governance

The Commission for Health Improvement (CHI) model of clinical governance draws on the same principles of clinical governance as the temple model and also illustrates that effective clinical governance is dependent upon an organisation being supportive of continuous learning, innovation and development. The CHI model shows the relationship between the patients' experience, the provider population's health and the organisation's capacity for improvement.

The CHI model of clinical governance (Commission for Health Improvement, 2001), envisages an organisation in which a 'strategic capacity' maps onto 'resources and processes' for achieving quality improvement. Both are underpinned by 'use of information' (Holloway, 2001). Organisational capacity is defined under the headings

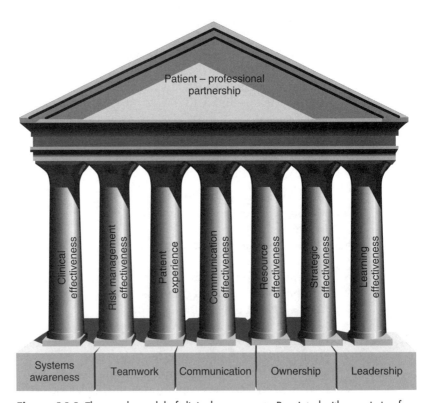

**Figure 14.1** The temple model of clinical governance. Reprinted with permission from www.cgsupport.nhs.uk.

'strategic capacity', 'resources and processes' and 'information', with a number of elements under each of these headings. Strategic capacity includes leadership, direction and planning, and patient focus, to emphasise the importance of leadership on strategy and on patients. Leaders must set the direction for the organisation and, if they do not focus on patients, then the organisation as a whole will lack that focus. Information about the patients' experience and health is critical to effective clinical governance and underpins the strategic capacity, resources and processes of an organisation (Commission for Health Improvement, 2001).

Application of the model leads to positive results for patients. The systems dictated by CHI for monitoring and improving services include: 'consultation and patient involvement; clinical risk management; clinical audit; research and effectiveness; staff training and staff management; education, training and continuing professional development; (and) the use of information about patients' experiences, outcomes and processes' (Commission for Health Improvement, 2001, p. xii).

## The Review, Agree, Implement, Develop/Demonstrate (RAID) model

The Review, Agree, Implement, Develop/Demonstrate (RAID) model is based on the quality cycle, first proposed by Deming in the 1950s as a systematic approach for businesses to adopt to continuously improve and respond to customers' needs (see Mann, 1989). In 1999, the NHS Clinical Governance Support Team was established to support the development and implementation of clinical governance (Halligan, 1999). As part of their work, they revised the RAID model of clinical governance. While other clinical governance models help to define what clinical governance is, and where attention needs paying to achieve high-quality health services, the RAID model of clinical governance (Figure 14.2) helps to embed clinical governance within an organisation, using four stages (Halligan & Donaldson, 2001):

(1) Review. A review of an organisation and its services that involves all stakeholders – staff, patients, health and local authorities, etc. – is carried out. This helps those implementing clinical governance to understand where the organisation is and how it is currently doing things. It identifies the visions and values of the organisation and examines the perceptions of stakeholders. The review process looks at all issues, including leadership, teamwork and communication. Reviews can also be carried out to make sure that clinical governance is recognised in smaller projects.

(2) Agree. Once the review has been carried out, widespread agreement is required about any changes that need to take place. Any necessary needs assessments should be carried out so that

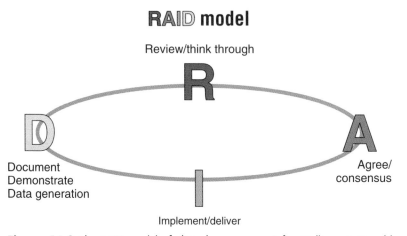

# RAID model

Review/think through

Document
Demonstrate
Data generation

Agree/
consensus

Implement/deliver

**Figure 14.2** The RAID model of clinical governance (after Halligan & Donaldson, 2001).

planning and preparation for implementation will take place. Ownership of any identified needs, and a commitment to making the changes happen, must be established.

(3) Implement. This stage brings about action by putting the agreed changes in place. This is carried out project-by-project, making sure that it happens successfully. Measuring success and identifying achievements and any further improvements that can be made are important components of implementation.

(4) Demonstrate and develop. This component of the RAID model is concerned with evaluation and measurement, which will ensure that improvements are ongoing and sustainable. This phase also examines the lessons that have been learnt; how good practice should be shared and how learning should take place across the organisation.

## The Plan, Do, Study and Act (PDSA) model

The Plan, Do, Study and Act (PDSA) model has been adopted by many NHS organisations. The aim of the model is to encourage constant change, reflection and demonstrable improvement. It recognises the dynamic nature of quality improvement, and how we learn from experience and feedback (Cleghorn & Headrick, 1996). It is a quick and simple model for testing new ideas to improve the quality of care, as illustrated in Figure 14.3.

The first phase of planning sets objectives and asks questions in an attempt to predict the kinds of change that are necessary. The 'Do'

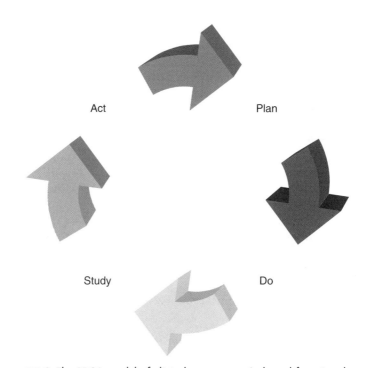

Act                                                    Plan

Study                                                  Do

**Figure 14.3** The PDSA model of clinical governance (adapted from Langley *et al.*, 1992).

phase is about carrying out the plan, documenting problems and unexpected observations and starting to analyse the data. 'Studying' completes this analysis, compares the data to predictions and makes a summary of the resultant learning. 'Act' makes the changes and prepares for starting the cycle again.

## Implementing clinical governance

Clinical governance recognises the importance of teams, organisations and systems in health care, rather than individuals working on their own (Halligan, 2003). The implementation and delivery of clinical governance includes the development of leadership, strategic planning for quality, patient involvement, information and analysis, staff and process management (Halligan & Donaldson, 2001). All of these must be achieved at an organisational level, but require the input of the organisation's most valuable resource – its staff – to do so (Harrison & Dixon, 2000). Organisations that empower their leaders, for example, will know how the vision, values and methods of clinical governance are being communicated effectively to all staff. 'Effective leadership empowers teamwork, creates an open and questioning culture, and ensures that both the ethos and the day-to-day delivery of clinical governance remain an integral part of every clinical service' (Halligan & Donaldson, 2001, p. 1414).

Clinical governance is primarily concerned with building a consistently safer and better NHS for patients. This means that, wherever possible, evidence-based practice should be in day-to-day use (Department of Health, 1997). Ensuring that patients receive high-quality care also means involving them in their own care. This is emphasised in a range of government policies and publications such as *A First Class Service* (Department of Health, 1998), *Making a Difference* (Department of Health, 1999c) and *The NHS Plan* (Department of Health, 2000b). A real partnership between patients and healthcare professionals is essential for effective clinical governance (Nichols *et al.*, 2000). It is important that clear systems are in place to enable information and feedback from patients to inform service development. Furthermore, empowering patients with information, and increasing their contribution to planning services, can greatly influence the development of clinical governance (Halligan & Donaldson, 2001).

## Ensuring effective systems

It is important to understand how processes for delivering healthcare services are designed to meet patient, quality and operational requirements (Halligan & Donaldson, 2001). Clinical governance places an emphasis on the identification of the potential risks in a situation, including the structures, relationships and systems involved in the delivery of health care, rather than fault finding. It identifies what works well, what does not work well and what needs improvement. Providing health care comes with risks for patients, for healthcare providers and for organisations. Risk management is a system that helps to minimise these risks. Minimising risks of injury or illness as a result of the way that health care is provided is vital.

It would be unrealistic to think that any healthcare system could be completely free of adverse healthcare events. Adverse healthcare events – an event or omission arising during clinical care and causing physical or psychological injury to a patient (Department of Health, 2000a) – happen in the NHS. While the frequency of these is relatively low, compared to the amount of care provided by the NHS, they do happen. When they do happen these events can be devastating for patients and their families, as well as for the staff involved. Patients suffer increased pain, disability and psychological trauma and staff can experience shame, guilt and depression. A report from the Department of Health (2000a) showed that adverse events take place in about 10% of admissions and cost £2 billion a year, that 400 people die or are seriously injured in adverse events and £400 million is paid out in clinical negligence claims every year. As well as adverse events, near misses –

situations in which an event or sequence of events or omissions arising during clinical care fails to develop further, thus preventing injury to the patient (Department of Health, 2000a) – also happen in the NHS.

To be effective, risk management needs to be supported by other systems, such as effective reporting mechanisms and complaints procedures. It also requires a blame-free culture that encourages staff to think that accidents are possible and to take all possible measures to prevent them from happening in the first place (Halligan & Donaldson, 2001). When they do happen – and mistakes do happen – it is essential that staff are able to report them without fear of reprisal. These elements are essential if problems are to be identified, evaluated, learned from and addressed. Equally, however, it is important that there are systems in place to deal with poor practitioner performance (Department of Health, 1999d). Learning effectively from adverse events and errors (Department of Health, 2000a) forms a part of clinical governance structures to improve the safety of the clinical environment.

## Complaints procedures

All NHS organisations are obliged to have a system to handle complaints, so that the complaint itself can be addressed, lessons can be learnt about what happened, and changes, where appropriate, can be made. In the NHS, complaints procedures encourage patients to complain directly to a NHS member of staff (Department of Health, 2004). Normally, complaints are dealt with by senior members of staff who have knowledge of the way complaints are dealt with, and who are able to deal with these quickly. It is often the case that complaints can be addressed on the spot and no further action or complaint is required. If further action is required, and a formal complaint is made, the complainant (normally a patient or his/her relatives) should receive a reply to their complaint within 20 days (Department of Health, 2004). If this does not adequately address their complaint, they can then complain to the complaints manager for the Trust. This may lead to a local review, which can include an independent panel and, in some cases, the patient's community health council. If patients are still unhappy with the response to their complaint, they can ask the Healthcare Commission for an 'Independent Review' of their case. The Healthcare Commission is an independent body established to promote improvements in health care. If they remain unsatisfied after this, they can complain to the Health Service Ombudsman. The Ombudsman is completely independent of the NHS and government (Department of Health, 2004).

## Patient services

The introduction of patient liaison services (PALS), in *The NHS Plan* (Department of Health, 2000b), means that every NHS organisation now has a key member of staff to support patients and carers with complaints. PALS are not part of the complaints procedure itself, but they offer advice and provide information about the complaints procedure and independent complaints advocacy services. PALS ensures that patients have support when things are going wrong, rather than just after the event, and means that some complaints can be handled and resolved on the spot.

While PALS acts locally in NHS Trusts, the National Patient Safety Agency (NPSA), established in July 2001, records and reviews systems to improve patient safety across the NHS. It collects and analyses patient safety information and provides feedback to healthcare organisations, staff, patients and carers in order to reduce future risk and to promote learning that will result in changes, where necessary, and quality improvement.

---

**Activity**

Can you think of an adverse event or near miss that has happened in your place of work?

- How was this dealt with?
- What has been learnt from this?
- Have changes been made as a result of the event?

---

## Support for the implementation of clinical governance

Several bodies have been established to ensure that clinical governance is being implemented. This includes the Health Care Commission, which replaced the work of the CHI, which carries out clinical governance reviews of all trusts, including acute, primary care, NHS Direct and ambulance trusts. A number of national standards are produced to ensure that the principles of clinical governance are applied to practice. The most commonly known of these are National Service Frameworks (NSFs) and clinical guidelines. These aim to ensure that health care is:

- based on best evidence
- delivered in the most effective way
- consistent.

### National Service Frameworks

*The NHS Plan* (Department of Health, 2000b) re-emphasised the role of NSFs as drivers in delivering the modernisation agenda. NSFs are long-term strategies for improving specific areas of care. The National

Service Framework for Coronary Heart Disease (Department of Health, 2000c), for example, states that 80% of patients who have a myocardial infarction should be prescribed aspirin, a beta blocker and statin therapy.

Each NSF is developed with an external reference group (ERG), which includes health professionals, service users and carers, health service managers, partner agencies and other advocates. They:

- set measurable goals to be delivered within set time frames
- set national standards and identify key interventions for a defined service or care group
- put in place strategies to support implementation
- establish ways to ensure progress within an agreed time scale
- form one of a range of measures to raise quality and decrease variations in service.

---

**Activity**

- How many National Service Frameworks can you name?
- Are there any that are relevant to your area of practice?
- How are they implemented in your place of work?

---

## Clinical guidelines

The National Institute for Health and Clinical Excellence (NICE) and other organisations draw up clinical guidelines, which set national service standards, define service models for a specific service or care group, suggest strategies to support implementation and establish performance measures against which progress, within an agreed time scale, is measured. Clinical guidelines are recommendations on the most appropriate treatment and care of people with specific diseases and conditions, based on the best available evidence. The British Hypertension Society, for example, has collaborated with NICE to review their guidelines for the management of hypertension in adults in primary care. The new guidelines (National Institute for Health and Clinical Excellence, 2006) state that the aim of treatment is to reduce blood pressure to 140/90 mmHg or below.

Designed to help healthcare professionals assimilate, evaluate and implement current best practice, clinical guidelines are a method of bridging the gap between academic research and everyday practice (Scottish Intercollegiate Guidelines Network, 1999). There are two main sources of clinical guidelines: national and local guidelines. National clinical guidelines are published by professional and healthcare bodies. Box 14.1 provides examples of the main organisations that produce National Service Frameworks and clinical guidelines.

## Box 14.1 Organisations that produce National Service Frameworks (NSFs) and clinical guidelines.

*The National Institute for Health and Clinical Excellence (NICE)*: NICE (http://www.nice.org.uk/) is an independent organisation responsible for providing national guidance on the promotion of good health and the prevention and treatment of ill health. It produces three types of guidance:

- Clinical guidelines on the appropriate treatment and care of people with specific diseases and conditions within the NHS in England and Wales.
- Technology appraisals, which provide guidance on the use of new and existing medicines and treatments within the NHS in England and Wales.
- Interventional procedures, which provide guidance on whether interventional procedures used for diagnosis or treatment are safe enough and work well enough for routine use in England, Wales and Scotland.

They also provide some information on the implementation of guidelines.

*The Department of Health*: The Department of Health (http://www.dh.gov.uk/Home/fs/en) sets standards and guidelines and NSFs for care across the NHS, social care and public health. NSFs are long-term strategies for improving specific areas of care. They set national standards and identify key interventions for a defined service or care group and set measurable goals to be achieved within an agreed time scale. The Department of Health also provides guidance on the implementation of these standards, guidelines and NSFs.

*The Royal College of Nursing (RCN)*: As part of its clinical effectiveness work, the RCN develops national nurse-led guidelines. The RCN is also involved in informing the development of other guidelines, providing a nursing perspective through membership of steering groups. The RCN website (http://www.rcn.org.uk/) provides links to partner organisations.

*The Royal College of Physicians (RCP)*: The RCP works to improve standards by influencing clinical practice through the generation of guidelines and audits. The website (http://www.rcplondon.ac.uk/) includes all UK guidelines produced in the previous 5 years that are considered relevant to the RCP, and non-UK guidelines that are relevant to UK practice (older guidelines may be included if new evidence does not exist).

*National Electronic Library for Health (NeLH)*: The NeLH (http://www.nelh.nhs.uk/) provides healthcare professionals with information to support the delivery of evidence-based health care. It has links to a number of relevant organisations as well as to specialist and health libraries and to a guidelines finder, which provides an index to over 1200 UK guidelines with links to downloadable versions.

**Activity**

- Can you identify other guidelines that you use in clinical practice?
- Choose one of these and summarise the key points that influence the care you deliver.
- How do you measure the care you give against the guidelines for best practice?

Local clinical guidelines are normally produced to address specific healthcare issues not addressed by national guidelines. Developing valid guidelines requires considerable expertise and resources, which are often beyond the scope of healthcare practitioners. Wherever possible, it is recommended that existing guidelines, which have included a systematic and rigorous review of the available evidence, are adapted for local use. If no such guidelines exist and it is considered necessary to develop one, then it is important that as rigorous a method as possible is used within the resources available. The Royal College of Nursing states that monitoring standards of care helps nurses to: maintain and improve their standards of care, participate in multi-professional team working, raise the profile of good nursing care and confirm that good nursing care affects patient outcomes.

The increasing availability of published high-quality systematic reviews make the task of identifying best evidence somewhat easier. The number of systematic reviews on specific nursing topics is, however, limited. In developing a local guideline it is important to acknowledge any potential limitations that arise from the nature of the evidence upon which the guideline is based, or the methods used in developing the guideline (Fedder *et al.*, 1999).

Once a relevant guideline has been identified it should be appraised in order to assess its validity. National guidelines published by organisations such as NICE or the Scottish Intercollegiate Guidelines Network (SIGN) have gone through a rigorous process of development and validation. Adopting recommendations from guidelines of questionable validity may lead to ineffective use of resources, inappropriate care or even harm to patients (Fedder *et al.*, 1999).

## The cyclical nature of clinical governance: measuring performance

Perhaps one of the most challenging aspects of clinical governance is its cyclical nature. There is no definitive outcome or end result. Once improvements have been achieved, the process tends to be opened up to further scrutiny to ensure that improvement is continuous and ongoing. It is a never-ending cycle of continuous improvement (W. Edwards Deming, see Mann, 1989). There are several ways in which performance in the delivery of health care can be, and is, measured.

## Clinical audit

The 1989 White Paper *Working For Patients* defines audit as 'the systematic, quantifiable comparison of specific clinical practices against explicit current standards in order to identify opportunities to improve the quality of patient care' (Department of Health, 1989). The aim of clinical audit is to review the quality of care. This does not include the cost of providing it. Unlike research, which aims to identify best evidence for treatment, audit measures the gap between actual practice and best evidence. It should be a cyclical activity, which ensures ongoing quality improvement, review and practice refinement.

Audit is a critical review of the care a patient receives, including procedures for diagnosis and treatment, and the outcome from the patient's perspective. The information gained from this is compared against evidence-based standards, for example NICE guidelines, and changes should be made if the outcomes of the audit fail to meet these standards.

## Benchmarking

The successful implementation of clinical governance depends on best practice being recognised in one service and being passed on to another. This process can be carried out in a number of ways: by using benchmarking, by setting guidelines and monitoring their use, by using quality improvement models and by people keeping up to date on relevant professional issues. Benchmarking is also discussed in Chapter 5.

In *Making a Difference* (Department of Health, 1999c) benchmarking is described as 'a process through which best practice is identified and continuous improvement pursued through comparison and sharing'. It should be seen as part of the broader quality agenda and an integral part of making sure that clinical governance is embedded in any health service. Benchmarking can take place at national, local or organisational levels. It helps to identify a baseline for comparing performance and involves the continuous process of measuring products, services and practices against identical practices of other healthcare organisations and against established best evidence. It involves six phases:

- Phase 1: agree area of practice
- Phase 2: establish a comparison group
- Phase 3: agreeing best practice
- Phase 4: scoring and then re-scoring

- Phase 5: comparison and sharing
- Phase 6: dissemination of good practice.

In phase three, scoring can take the following form:

Worst practice                            Benchmark of best practice
<br>     E         D         C         B         A

Benchmarking is a good learning tool, because, by looking at how others work, it is possible to identify better ways of working that can be incorporated into your own practice. It is a tool that can be used to measure clinical effectiveness (see Chapter 15 for more information about clinical effectiveness).

## Summary

- The same level of safe, high-quality care should be available to all patients, regardless of where they live or who treats them.
- Patients should be at the centre of health care and therefore should inform its developments.
- There are a number of models of clinical governance, which can be used to develop and evaluate it.
- Setting, delivering and monitoring care and delivery standards help to ensure effective high-quality health care and embed clinical governance into healthcare.
- While clinical governance is an organisational issue, it is not possible without the input and participation of its staff.
- Ensuring that staff understand and are supported in the implementation of clinical governance is key to its success.

# References

Cleghorn, G D & Headrick, L A (1996) The PDSA cycle at the core of learning in health professions education. *Joint Commission Journal On Quality Improvement* 22 (3): 206–12.

Commission for Health Improvement (2001) *Report of a Clinical Governance Review at Northern Birmingham Mental Health NHS Trust.* Stationery Office, London.

Commission for Health Improvement (2002) *Report of a Clinical Governance Review at South London and Maudsley NHS Trust.* Stationery Office, London.

Department of Health (1989) *Working for Patients.* Stationery Office, London.

Department of Health (1997) White Paper. *The New NHS: Modern, Dependable.* Stationery Office, London.

Department of Health (1998) *A First Class Service. Quality in the NHS.* HMSO, London.

Department of Health (1999a) *The Health Act.* HMSO, London. Available at http://www.opsi.gov.uk/acts/acts1999/19990008.htm

Department of Health (1999b) *Clinical Governance in the New NHS.* HSC 1999/065, Department of Health, London.

Department of Health (1999c) *Making a Difference: Strengthening the Nursing, Midwifery and Health Visiting Contribution to Health and Healthcare.* HMSO, London.

Department of Health (1999d) *Supporting Doctors, Protecting Patients.* HMSO, London.

Department of Health (2000a) *An Organisation with a Memory: Report of an Expert Group on Learning from Adverse Events in the NHS Chaired by the Chief Medical Officer.* HMSO, London.

Department of Health (2000b) *The NHS Plan: A Plan for Investment, A Plan for Reform.* HMSO, London.

Department of Health (2000c) *National Service Framework for Coronary Heart Disease.* HMSO, London.

Department of Health (2004) *How to Make a Complaint about the NHS.* HMSO, London. http://www.dh.gov.uk/assetRoot/04/02/00/39/04020039. pdf

Fedder, G, Eccles, M, Grol, R, Griffiths, C & Grimshaw, J (1999) Clinical guidelines: using clinical guidelines. *British Medical Journal* 318: 728–30.

Hallet, L & Thompson, M (2000) *Clinical Governance: A Practical Guide for Managers.* Emap Public Sector Management, London.

Halligan, A (1999) How the national clinical governance support team plans to support the development of clinical governance in the workplace. *Journal of Clinical Governance* 7: 155–7.

Halligan, A (2003) The implementation of clinical governance. *Health Director* Mar/Apr: 14–15.

Halligan, A & Donaldson, L (2001) Implementing clinical governance: turning vision into reality. *British Medical Journal* 322: 1413–17.

Harrison, A & Dixon, J (2000) *The NHS Facing the Future.* Kings Fund, London.

Holloway, F (2001) The inspector calls. The CHI comes to town. *The Psychiatric Bulletin* 25: 457–8.

Langley, G J, Nolan, K M & Nolan, T W (1992) *The Foundation Improvement.* API Publishing, Silver Spring, MD.

Mann, N R (1989) *The Keys to Excellence – The Deming Philosophy.* Mercury, London.

National Institute for Health and Clinical Excellence (2006) *Hypertension: Management of Hypertension in Adults in Primary Care: Partial Update.* Royal College of Physicians, London. Available at www.nice.org.uk/ CG034

Nichols, S, Cullen, R, O'Neill, S & Halligan A (2000) Clinical governance: its origins and its foundations. *Clinical Performance and Quality Health Care* 8 (3): 172–8.

Scally, G & Donaldson, L J (1998) Clinical governance and the drive for quality improvement in the new NHS in England. *British Medical Journal* 317: 61–5.

Scottish Intercollegiate Guidelines Network (1999) *SIGN Guidelines: An Introduction to SIGN Methodology for the Development of Evidence Based Clinical Guidelines.* SIGN Publication No. 39. SIGN Secretariat, Edinburgh.

# Practice development and clinical effectiveness

**15**

## Learning objectives

- Understand the principles of change and how they can be used effectively in the healthcare setting.
- Understand what practice development is and how it can used to provide high-quality health care.
- Understand what clinical effectiveness means and the importance of delivering clinically effective high-quality care.
- Identify ways practice development and clinical effectiveness can improve patient care.

## Introduction

In this chapter the principles of changing practice to improve the quality of care will be discussed in the context of healthcare delivery. Practice development and clinical effectiveness will be defined and ways of disseminating best practice discussed.

In recent years, health and social care reforms have focused on improving the quality of clinical practice and patient care. There are several reasons for this, which include a rise in public expectations of the NHS, increased availability of health information and an acknowledgement that healthcare provision could be improved (Department of Health, 2000). In every generation of health care there have been practices that have subsequently been shown to be ineffective (Clifford & Clark, 2004). The challenge for nurses is not only to deliver the best possible care to patients, but also to be able to clearly demonstrate that they do so.

An essential role of all nurses is to deliver high-quality health care, but what is meant by quality of care?

---

**Activity**

Think of what quality of care means to you.

- How do you know if you are providing high-quality health care?
- Ask your friends and family what quality of care means to them.
- Are their views different to your own ideas about quality of care?

---

Quality in health care is an all-encompassing term that includes: carrying out a job to the best of your ability; practice that is based on evidence; putting research into practice; setting and maintaining standards of care; writing and following protocols, procedures and policies which are based on best practice; and continually questioning practice to ensure that the best care possible is provided. There are many definitions of quality of care, which are dependent on the context in which they are being used. Reeves & Bednar (1994) assert that a global definition for quality does not exist, and there are different definitions of quality that are appropriate in differing circumstances. Tuchman (1980, p. 38) defines quality in relation to excellence:

> *Quality means investment of the best skill and effort possible to produce the finest and most admirable results possible . . . Quality is achieving or reaching for the highest standard.*

Whereas Ovretveit (1992, p. 14) defines quality in terms of efficiency as:

> *Fully meeting the needs of those who need the service most, at the lowest cost to the organisation within the limits and directives set by higher authorities and purchasers.*

## Change

Change may be defined as an attempt to alter or replace existing knowledge, skills, attitudes and styles of individuals and groups (Wright, 1989). The facilitation of change is fundamental to improving the quality of care. In order to be able to bring about change in practice it is important to have an understanding of the process of change. Change is a dynamic process that is necessary to enable continuous improvement in the delivery of patient care.

The first step in the process of improving the quality of care is to think about current practice and to determine whether it is the most effective care, based on the best evidence available. This process is described in Chapter 11.

## Change theory

There are a number of theories of change. Many of these have their roots in the work of Lewin (1951), who described the process of successful change in three stages:

(1) *Unfreezing*: where the need for change is recognised. At this stage professionals should be encouraged, supported and motivated in the direction of the desired change through an introduction to the (new) evidence and involvement in the process of change.
(2) *Movement*: where the change process gets under way. Familiarisation with the (new) evidence results in an alteration in beliefs and behaviour so that desired change(s) begin to take place.
(3) *Refreezing*: where there is an acceptance and integration of the change. The new behaviour(s) and belief(s) become the professionals' 'own'. At this stage encouragement through positive feedback and support are important in order that change is achieved and maintained.

In order to effect change there are a number of strategies that can be used. Haffer (1986) describes three strategies, which are commonly used to effect change:

(1) *The power coercive approach*: this is known as a 'top-down' approach and is used in a hierarchical manner. It can bring about rapid change, but is often met with resistance, making permanent and effective change difficult.
(2) *The empirical rational approach*: this is also a 'top-down' approach. It assumes that the majority of individuals are rational and that they will comply, but does not account for those individuals who are not used to taking orders.
(3) *The normative re-educative approach*: this is a 'bottom-up' participative approach and is the most democratic of the approaches. It is based on the belief that everyone affected by a change should be involved in it. Any changes are likely to be long lasting; however, it is very time consuming and difficult for individuals who are used to taking orders.

The NHS is changing at a rapid pace. In order to achieve successful change an organisation needs its members to be adaptable. Ford (1997) argues that ideally change should be viewed as necessary rather than inevitable, and that staff are less likely to be conducive to change if they do not see the need for it. A rapid pace of change can cause low morale, a drop in productivity, narrow outlook and reluctance to take risks. Due to insecurities brought about by change, it is not always thought to be positive by those affected by it. It is important to recognise this when attempting to bring about a change and to remember that individuals may feel threatened by change, especially if they have been carrying out a particular practice for a long time.

It is important to remember that before you begin something new you have to end what was there before. However, the process of change is not that simple, there has to be a transition period. People do not tend to like endings and it is important that the loss that some individuals feel is acknowledged. Often the ending of practice can imply criticism, a sense that what was being done previously was wrong. This, coupled with the fact that people do not like to stop doing things that they have been doing for a long time, is often the cause of misunderstanding and resistance to change.

## Practice development and clinical effectiveness

A number of systems have been introduced into the NHS to support the development of quality and continuous improvement in health care. Two major concepts that address this are practice development and clinical effectiveness. While both of these focus on methods of improving the quality of care, practice development is concerned with the broader issues involved in the process of care delivery and clinical effectiveness is concerned with specific interventions within that process.

## Practice development

### What is practice development?

Practice development is about creating an environment of excellence in care, which puts the patient at the centre of all that nurses, as health professionals, do.

---

**Activity**

- In what ways do you think this can be achieved?
- Can you think of examples of practice development that you have achieved?

---

The practice development agenda in health care in general, and more specifically in nursing, is gaining strength and credibility, and is becoming an increasingly important role in healthcare delivery. Practice development ensures that the most appropriate care is given to patients by ensuring that health care is delivered in the best possible way and that there are systems in place to support and sustain this good practice. It is important to utilise best evidence to deliver best practice (the importance of evidence-based practice is discussed in Chapter 11).

Practice development does not have a beginning or an end, it is a continuous process of growth and improvement. It is a way of practising that, once fostered, evolves, often having a 'knock-on effect' on the systems of care. Practice development can lead to improved quality and excellence in care, which benefits patients, practitioners and organisations. It is a way of enabling both individuals and teams to deliver innovative, patient-centred care (Page, 2002).

One popular definition of practice development is that of Garbett & McCormack (2002, p. 88), who define practice development as:

> *A continuous process of improvement towards increased effectiveness in patient centred care. This is brought about by helping health care teams to develop their knowledge and skills to transform the culture and context of care. It is enabled and supported by facilitators committed to systematic rigorous continuous processes of emancipatory change that reflect the perspectives of service users.*

There are a number of sources of information on practice development that can be used to gain more understanding about its application. The Royal College of Nursing (RCN), for example, has developed a designated practice development area within their members' website (http://www.rcn.org.uk/resources/practicedevelopment/index.php). The RCN defines practice development as being:

> *... designed to help you approach your work in new ways by helping you to: offer better choices for patients; provide evidence-based and patient centred care; challenge and reflect on the care that you provide; recognise and overcome obstacles that limit your ability to deliver best care; sustain yourself and your team to continue with learning and positive change; demonstrate the impact you have on practice; influence and shape social policy.*

Whichever definition of practice development is most appropriate to your own practice, it is clear that it is rapidly becoming an essential part of any healthcare organisation's short-, medium and long-term policy (McSherry & Bassett, 2002).

In general, the aims of practice development are to:

- create an environment of excellence in care
- place the patient at the centre
- utilise best evidence to deliver best practice
- create a motivated and adaptable healthcare workforce.

Practice development provides a way of improving the quality of services. It encourages collaborative partnerships and provides a network for sharing. It must be remembered that practice development is part of all nurses' roles. While practice development differs from one organisation to another, it is increasingly considered essential for both modernising health care and for improving the quality of health care. Practice development can be achieved through the facilitation of change, encouraging collaborative partnerships and providing a network of sharing and disseminating information.

## Why is practice development important?

Documents such as *A First Class Service* (Department of Health, 1998), *Making a Difference* (Department of Health, 1999) and *The NHS Plan* (Department of Health, 2000) stress that in order to address the challenges of healthcare delivery in the twenty-first century the NHS needs to change. This change in focus to continuous improvement in health care is one of the primary reasons that practice development has moved to the forefront of healthcare delivery, rather than being seen as separate and optional to it.

Fish (1998) argued that research and practice development were not always seen as inherent parts of healthcare practice, even though they are central to the ability of a profession to define its own knowledge base. More recently, they have become a recognised part of healthcare delivery, which is essential not only in ensuring the delivery of quality of care, but also in ensuring that there is a continuous improvement of that health care. While there was once ambivalence about the responsibility and opportunity to develop care (Kitchen, 1997), practitioners are increasingly responsible for developing care as well as delivering it. McSherry & Bassett (2002) stated that practice development is about the integration of research-based evidence into health care. In practice it is more than that. It includes influencing change by putting evidence into practice, and meeting the needs of patients, practitioners and organisations in the presence or absence of research based evidence.

## How can practice development be achieved?

The application of best evidence in practice by practitioners is fundamental to achieving practice development. There are several national and local tools to support this. National tools include a number of organisations that influence the standards of the delivery of health care:

- *National Institute for Health and Clinical Excellence* (http://www.nice.org.uk/): guidance about what to do (and sometimes what not to do).
- *National Patient Safety Agency* (http://www.npsa.nhs.uk/): making the NHS safer for patients.
- *National Clinical Assessment Authority* (http://www.ncaa.nhs.uk/): helps local organisations with the assessment of doctors whose performance gives concern.
- *The Healthcare Commission* (http://www.healthcarecommission.org.uk/): the independent watch dog that reports to Parliament on the performance of Trusts in England and Wales.

---

**Activity**

- What processes do you know of that support the development of practice?
- What do you think your role is in the development of practice?

---

Achieving practice development at the local level can include the use of the following:

- Clinical governance: the *Research Governance Framework for Health and Social Care* (Department of Health, 2001) defines this as aiming to continually improve the overall standards of clinical care in the NHS and to reduce unacceptable variations in clinical practice.
- Clinical audit: the primary goal of clinical audit should be to foster a climate in which healthcare professionals collaborate to provide the highest quality of health care possible (Lugon & Secker-Walker, 1999).
- Organisational development: provides a system for managing change, which can help make improvements happen.

It is useful when starting any practice development project to review the current situation first. Figure 15.1 outlines some of the questions that should be addressed before the commencement of the project.

It is important to focus on the positive rather than the negative in order to motivate teams. Questions like these are useful:

| | |
|---|---|
| • What is excellent? | • What is bad? |
| • What is good?    *Rather than* | |
| • What could be better? | • What are we doing wrong? |
| • What is unsafe? | |

Spelling out the issues for change and providing clear guidance through effective communication are important in achieving change through practice development.

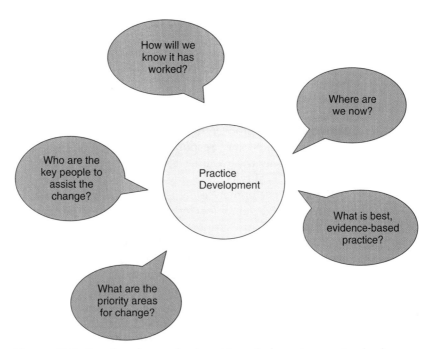

**Figure 15.1** Questions that need to be addressed when using practice development to improve care.

---

**Activity**

Imagine that you are working in an area where you have identified a need for a change in practice.

- How will you go about achieving that change?
- What is it that you will need to consider?

Using the checklist below, work through the steps you will need to take to make change happen.

- Why do you consider it to be important?
- Who else considers it to be important?
  **Hint**: colleagues/patients/research
- Who will benefit from the change?
- What will the benefits be?
  **Hint:** efficiency, effectiveness, quality of life
- What are the arguments to justify your need for change?
- What processes can be put in place to assist with the change?
  **Hint**: training, information, organisation change
- Who do you need to work with to change the practice?
- Who/what are the potential barriers to the change?
- What resources do you need to achieve the change?
- What skills do you need to achieve the change?

## *Practice development nurses*

Many healthcare organisations, and in particular the NHS, have recognised the importance of achieving change in practice and have employed practice development nurses specifically for this role. Some organisations have posts where the whole of the job is devoted to practice development; however, increasingly many posts are being developed with practice development as an aspect of the role. While job descriptions and responsibilities vary between organisations, key roles generally include leadership, education and training, and quality.

Practice development is achieved through the facilitation of innovation and the development of evidence-based nursing. Leadership is essential in order to support ward, department and community-based practitioners in the planning and implementation of practice development, which may lead to the implementation of changes to nursing roles and practice. Practice development plays a leading role in the production and implementation of evidence-based guidelines and protocols, and also in the setting, delivery and sustainability of high standards. The provision of support to managers in the delivery of clinical governance processes assures the quality of the fundamental aspects of patient care.

Practice development involves the development and implementation of educational programmes and provision of an environment that supports learning. This includes a continuous professional development programme, which reflects the current NHS research and development agenda. Practice development also has a role in ensuring clinical placements meet the requirements of nurse training and education, and links with Practice Placement Facilitators and Higher Education Institutes are important in influencing the curriculum for new nurses.

# Clinical effectiveness

## *What is clinical effectiveness?*

Clinical effectiveness is about doing the right thing in the right way and at the right time for the right patient (Royal College of Nursing, 1996). This means that practitioners have to examine systematically everything they do in caring for patients, in order to make sure that they are providing beneficial care and not wasting staff and patients' time, resources and public monies by providing services that do not actually help patients (NHS Executive, 1996).

Clinical effectiveness has three main functions (NHS Executive, 1996):

- being sure that everyone knows what clinically effective practice is
- applying knowledge about clinically effective practice in day-to-day patient care
- making sure that changes in practice are working to benefit patients.

It is important that all nurses understand the meaning of clinical effectiveness and have access to the best possible evidence about the care they provide. All nurses need to be able to utilise the available evidence in their everyday working practices to influence changes in care. It is necessary for nurses to work collaboratively with other professionals in order to achieve this. It is almost impossible for a lone individual to implement sustainable change. Successful change requires the support and engagement of colleagues, and any changes made to care provision need to have a positive impact on the care of patients. It is also important to have systems in place to monitor the effect or impact of changes in practice, for example through carrying out clinical audit or research.

Clinical effectiveness is an ongoing process. Figure 15.2 demonstrates the cyclical nature of this process.

---

**Activity**

Think about the area of practice in which you work.

- Are you certain that you are delivering best practice?
- Is your practice based on research findings?
- Is your practice based on expert opinion?
- Do you have clinical guidelines/standards that you work to?
- Have you or your colleagues discussed and agreed on best practice?
- Has a clinical audit been carried out to confirm that you are following best practice?
- Is there a need to make improvements?
- Can you think of ways to ensure practice is clinically effective?

---

## Why is clinical effectiveness important?

There are many benefits to providing care that is clinically effective. Patients who receive care that is clinically effective will have better healthcare outcomes. This means that they recover more quickly and receive better care. Less time will be wasted on care that is less beneficial and this may lead to shorter stays in hospital or less time attending

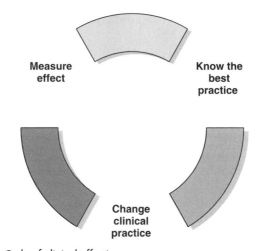

**Figure 15.2** Cycle of clinical effectiveness.

for appointments. If all nurses are delivering care to the same best practice standards, this will also mean that patients will have more consistent care. This may lead to patients being more satisfied with their care and more confident about the healthcare system.

Collaborative and consistent working practices benefit all individuals within the multi-professional team. For nurses the importance of taking responsibility for clinical effectiveness, regardless of their position in the team, is essential. It is important to remember the Nursing and Midwifery Council's *Code of Professional Conduct* (2002), section 6.5, which states:

> *As a registered nurse, midwife or health visitor, you must maintain your professional knowledge and competence. You have a responsibility to deliver care based on current evidence, best practice and, where applicable, validated research when it is available.*

Contributing to the delivery of the most appropriate and effective care available within a dynamic and supportive team is satisfying and rewarding. Constantly examining and assessing practice ensures that clinical effectiveness is achieved and sustained. Clinically effective practices also ensure that the risk(s) of causing harm to patients is reduced and that care is more cost effective.

## *How does clinical effectiveness work?*

This chapter has discussed the way in which evidence can be put into practice and that, at its best, clinical effectiveness is the implementation of best evidence to ensure the best possible care for patients. One of the ongoing difficulties in healthcare delivery is that much of the day-to-day care that nurses carry out for patients is not supported by evidence. It can be difficult to know what to do in these situations. There are, however, a number of ways in which to ensure clinical effectiveness in patient care with or without the existence of evidence.

If there is no current best evidence available, one way to be clinically effective is to find out what the experts recommend as best practice. This method will ensure that the best practice guidance comes from experts in the area or field and their recommendations can be adopted. This usually involves canvassing a number of experts in that particular field across the country and collating expert opinion. A consensus of the opinion of experts may be the best option in the absence of valid research, for example. Another useful method of finding out what is clinically effective care is to seek advice from national, regional or local resource centres. There are many organisations (for example The Stroke Association, Action on Epilepsy, Diabetes UK) who produce guidance on best practice for their particular area of expertise (see Chapter 11 for more discussion on finding best evidence).

Finally, when there is no other evidence available or groups to consult for advice, it is possible to reach a consensus with other experienced nursing and other professional colleagues on best practice and agree an effective way to provide care.

## Outcomes

The outcomes of practice development and clinical effectiveness are improved patient experiences and outcomes. In workplaces where staff at all levels understand their responsibility, high-quality clinically effective care and the ongoing development of practice takes place. The ultimate outcome is a continued improvement of the quality of care, with sustainable change in practice to ensure that best practice is delivered. It is not necessarily a 'project' with neatly defined start and end dates (Clark & Proctor, 1999). Successful outcomes include:

- improvement in the quality of care
- evidence-based practice
- standardisation of best care.

Binnie & Titchen (1999) found that having a patient-centred philosophy is central to promoting and supporting the 'right' kind of practice. Practice which is explicitly evidence-based and patient focused can be achieved through practice development and clinical effectiveness.

**Summary**

- Change management strategies can be used to ensure that best practice is achieved and sustained.
- Practice development can lead to improved quality and excellence in care, which benefits patients, practitioners and organisations.
- Clinical effectiveness enables nurses to reflect on why they do what they do for patients and to systematically find and implement better ways of caring for patients.

# References

Binnie, A & Titchen, A (1999) *Freedom to Practise: The Development of Patient Centred Nursing.* Butterworth Heinemann, London.

Clark, C & Proctor, S (1999) Practice development: ambiguity in research and practice. *Journal of Advanced Nursing* 30 (4): 975–82.

Clifford, C & Clark, J (2004) *Getting Research into Practice.* Churchill Livingstone, London.

Department of Health (1998) *A First Class Service: Quality in the New NHS.* The Stationery Office, London.

Department of Health (1999) *Making a Difference: Strengthening the Nursing Midwifery and Health Visiting Contribution to Health and Healthcare.* The Stationery Office, London.

Department of Health (2000) *The NHS Plan: A Plan for Investment, A Plan for Reform.* The Stationery Office, London.

Department of Health (2001) *Research Governance Framework for Health and Social Care.* The Stationery Office, London.

Fish, D (1998) *Appreciating Practice and the Caring Professions – Refocussing Professional Development and Practitioner Research.* Butterworth Heinemann, Oxford.

Ford, S (1997) Change? No problem. *Nursing Management* 4 (5): 12–14.

Garbett, R & McCormack, B (2002) A concept analysis of practice development. *NT Research* 7 (2): 87–100.

Haffer, A (1986) Facilitating change: choosing the appropriate strategy. *Journal of Nursing Administration* 16 (4): 18–22.

Kitchen, S S (1997) Research, the therapist and the patient. *Journal of Interprofessional Care* 11 (1): 49–55.

Lewin, K (1951) *Field Theory and Social Sciences.* Harper & Row, New York.

Lugon, M & Secker-Walker, J (1999) *Clinical Governance: Making it Happen.* The Royal Society of Medicine Press, Cardiff.

McSherry, R & Bassett, C (2002) *Practice Development in the Clinical Setting: A Guide to Implementation.* Nelson Thornes, London.

NHS Executive (1996) *Clinical Effectiveness – What's it All About?* NHS Executive, Leeds.

Nursing and Midwifery Council (2002) *Code of Professional Conduct.* NMC, London.

Ovretveit, J (1992) *Health Service Quality.* Blackwell Scientific Publications, London.

Page, S (2002) The role of practice development in modernising the NHS. *Nursing Times* 98 (11): 34–6.

Reeves, C A & Bednar, D A (1994) Defining quality: Alternatives and implications. *Academy of Management Review* 19 (3): 419–46.

Royal College of Nursing (1996) *Clinical Effectiveness. A Royal College of Nursing Guide.* RCN, London.

Tuchman, B W (1980) The decline of quality. *New York Times Magazine* 2 (104): 38–41.

UKCC (United Kingdom Central Council for Nursing, Midwifery and Health Visiting) (1992) *The Scope of Professional Practice.* UKCC, London.

Wright, S (1989) *Changing Nursing Practice.* Edward Arnold, London.

# Scope of professional practice

16

## Learning objectives

- Understand how and why the roles of nurses and other health-care professionals have developed.
- Demonstrate an understanding of how nurses and others develop their knowledge and identify the differences between a novice and expert practitioner.
- Understand how reflection is carried out and how it can inform changes to, and the development of, clinical practice.
- Be aware of the role that professional regulation plays in the development and maintenance of standards of health care.
- Understand how current and ongoing developments have affected the role of nurses and other healthcare professionals and the implications of this for professional regulation.

## Introduction

This chapter will discuss the development of nursing as a profession and the development of nursing practice. This will include a discussion of the scope of professional practice and the development of registered nurses as well as those allied to nursing, such as auxiliaries and health-care assistants. It will include, as part of this, a consideration of the legislation and professional regulation of practice, as well as the development of roles. At a more fundamental level it considers how nurses and those who work with them develop their knowledge and skills, from that of novice to expert practitioners. It also considers the role of reflection in this process through the development of insight and changes to practice.

Challenges to health service delivery, which include increases in chronic and long-term illness, growing demands for efficiency and effectiveness, changes in patients' expectations, and a reduction in junior doctors' hours, have led to a consideration of the way in which health services are configured. As a result, many organisations have reoriented and integrated their workforce across occupations and disciplines to more effectively utilise the skills and roles required to meet service needs (Buchan, 2002). Ultimately, they seek 'smarter' ways of working.

Service managers support a multi-disciplinary approach as a means of meeting these ever-increasing demands in organisations where performance is increasingly measured in terms of economy and efficiency. Leaders in nursing view the promotion of a multi-disciplinary approach to patient care as part of the continued professional development of nursing. Nurses have taken on more of the work traditionally undertaken by doctors. The development of nursing practice presents numerous implications in clinical practice. It requires nurses to develop their ways of thinking about and handling clinical practice.

## The development of the nursing profession

Nursing has a long-established tradition of caring and compassion, intuition and empathy (Davies, 1995). Florence Nightingale's (1865) contention that to be a good nurse, one must be a good woman reflects the Victorian values that have surrounded the development of nursing. The medical community vigorously protested the education of nursing in the university setting, and plans to train 'lady nurses' at St Thomas and Guys Hospitals in 1860 met with resistance from the medical profession, who would not sanction a nursing system that was not under their direct control (Peterson, 1978). In 1908 Dr W. Gilman Thompson summarised the attitude of most physicians at the time, stating:

> *Nursing is not, strictly speaking, a profession. A profession implies . . . attainments in special knowledge as distinguished from mere skill . . . (nursing) is not primarily designed to contribute to the sum of human knowledge or the advancement of science. The great and principle duty of a nurse is to make a patient comfortable in bed, something not always attained by the most bookish of nurse. Any intelligent, not necessarily educated woman can in a short time acquire the skill to carry out with implicit obedience the physician's directions* (Thompson, 1906, p. 846).

In the first half of the twentieth century, medical education moved rapidly into the university setting. Nursing education, however, remained solidly linked to hospital administration through the labour of nursing students. Medicine controlled the social and economic power of nursing. It incorporated principles of physiology, microbiology, chemistry, bacteriology, immunology and even psychology into the domain of medical knowledge. In contrast, nursing was seen as an extension of the maternal role. It had no legitimate claim to scientific knowledge, the exclusive realm of men and, in particular, doctors. Power relations between (male) doctors and (female) nurses was epitomised in the notion that nurses were to be 'trained' while doctors were to be 'educated' (Doering, 1992). Florence Nightingale's view (Nightingale, 1865, p. 14) that it was 'the duty of the medical officer to give what orders, in regard to the sick, he thinks fit to the nurses. And . . . unquestionably the duty of the nurses to obey or to see his orders are carried out' reinforced this view.

Since the 1970s nursing has attempted to reconstruct itself as an independent profession. Henderson (1969) and Rogers (1970), who were influential in nursing at that time, clearly distinguished the role of nursing from that of the doctor's assistant in their definitions of nursing. Nursing is emerging as an integral part of the health service. This presents numerous implications in relation to the roles of nurses in clinical practice, with the most important, perhaps, the demands of increased professional responsibility.

---

**Activity**

Consider the discussion above.

- Do you think that traditional views of the nurse as a female, who carries out doctors' orders, have completely disappeared from current perceptions about the role of the nurse?

Think about this in relation to your current role.

---

## Scope of practice and professional standards

The advancement of health care in general has influenced unprecedented changes in care delivery and provided nursing with the opportunity to develop and expand. The past 6 years, in particular, have seen considerable development in nursing roles in the UK. Nursing has risen to the challenges presented by both the UK government and the expectations of twenty-first-century health care. Nursing is a complex and rapidly changing profession that is demanding nurses who assume roles with advanced skills and knowledge (Higgins, 2003). Changes to professional roles, which include the freedom of nurses to practise more autonomously, have been accompanied by increased professional accountability for the decisions that they make in practice.

Accountability and responsibility are often used interchangeably and it is important to distinguish between the two. Responsibility implies answerability; it entails the ability of the individual to 'choose one course of action or intervention over another' as the correct choice in a given set of circumstances (Holden, 1991, p. 398). In contrast, accountability presents a sense of overriding concern for the whole process of decision making as it 'entails both personal and professional responsibility' (Holden, 1991, p. 398). Thus, while accountability requires responsibility, responsibility does not require accountability. Therefore, one may be held responsible, yet not accountable, for a decision or action. A common example of this taking place in clinical practice is through the delegation of patient care. While one nurse assumes responsibility for delivering patient care, the other, having delegated that care, is ultimately accountable for the care given (Harding & Grieg, 1994). This issue is particularly relevant today where delegation of care from doctors to nurses and from nurses to healthcare assistants is common.

---

**Activity**

Think about the way that care is organised in your place of work.

- Do you delegate care to others, or provide care that has been delegated to you?

Think about the implications of these situations in relation to responsibility and accountability.

- Do you know when you are responsible and when you are accountable for care?

---

## The Nursing and Midwifery Council

The Nursing and Midwifery Council (NMC) was established in April 2002 by Parliament when it took over from the former regulator: the United Kingdom Central Council for Nursing, Midwifery and Health Visiting (UKCC). The principle functions of the NMC are set out in legislation (*NMC Order*; Statutory Instrument, 2001) as follows:

- To establish standards of education
- To set up standards of training
- To set up standards of conduct

- To set up standards of performance
- To ensure the maintenance of those standards

In order that feelings of ambiguity regarding roles and role boundaries are reduced, professional bodies routinely adopt codes of conduct. Their principle function is to provide a point of reference upon which professional practice can be based. With its obligations in the improvement of professional conduct and in the protection of the public, amongst other roles, the NMC, the regulatory body for nurses and midwives in the UK, published a *Code of Professional Conduct* in 2002.

The *Code of Professional Conduct* (Nursing and Midwifery Council, 2002) provides the main source of professional accountability from the NMC. The 2002 edition revised previous versions published by the UKCC in 1983 and 1984. 'The Code' is introduced by the following statement: As a registered nurse or midwife, you are personally accountable for your practice. In caring for your patients and clients you must:

- respect the patient or client as an individual
- obtain consent before you give any treatment or care
- protect confidential information
- cooperate with others in the team
- maintain your professional knowledge and competence
- be trustworthy
- act to identify and minimise risk to all patients and clients.

These are the shared values of all the UK healthcare regulatory bodies.

It is apparent from the NMC's Code of Conduct that neither accountability or responsibility are optional extras in professional nursing practice. It includes references to the responsibilities of the nurse throughout its seven clauses.

Ongoing changes to roles in health care have placed unprecedented pressures on individuals taking on new roles. These pressures are not only in terms of accepting responsibility for the roles they assume, but also in terms of the learning and development required to be competent to do so. While some of the types of knowledge that affect professionals' decision making and competence were discussed in Chapter 10, the information below examines the ways in which this knowledge is gained. Both the 'Novice to Expert' model (Benner, 1984) and the process of reflection are discussed in relation to the development of professional knowledge and skills.

## Knowledge for practice

### *Novice to expert model*

The literature reveals numerous theories regarding the development of practical knowledge and skill. Perhaps the most widely known in nursing is that of the Model of Skill Acquisition (Benner, 1984). Origi-nally developed by Dreyfus & Dreyfus (1980), The Model of Skill Acquisition was applied to nursing by Patricia Benner (1984) and has been accepted by the majority of nurse educationalists and practitioners. The model implies that individuals progress in theory and practice according to their experience. It refers to the process of ongoing development as the nurse passes through five stages of development.

### Stage 1: Novice

The novice has no experience of the situations in which they are expected to perform. He/she learns to recognise various objects, facts and features relevant to the skill and acquires rules for determining actions based upon those facts and features. Both the elements of the situation that are relevant and the rules that are to be applied to these facts, regardless of what else is happening, are context free. Through information processing, the novice manipulates unambiguously defined, context free, elements by precise rules. The novice nurse, for example, is taught how to read blood pressure, measure bodily outputs and compute fluid balance, and is given rules for determining what to do when these measurements reach certain values (Dreyfus & Dreyfus, 1986).

The rule-governed behaviour of the novice is extremely limited and inflexible. Since they have no experience of the situations they encoun-ter, rules or protocols guide their performance. Rules, however, cannot inform the novice of the most relevant tasks to perform in a real situa-tion, and as a result, can legislate against successful performance (Benner, 1984). This point illustrates the situational and experience focus of the Dreyfus model, which distinguishes between the level of skilled performance that can be achieved through knowledge of prin-ciples and theory, and that which can be acquired in real situations (Dreyfus, 1982).

### Stage 2: Advanced beginner

Performance improves to a marginally acceptable level only after the novice has considerable experience in real situations. This experience enables the individual to note, or to have pointed out to him/her, the recurring meaningful situational components that are unique to real situations. Termed 'aspects of the situation' in the Dreyfus model, these, in contrast to the measurable, context-free attributes learned and used by the beginner, include overall global characteristics that can be identified only through prior experience (Benner, 1984). Rules for behaviour now refer to both situational and context-free components. For example, the nurse at this stage learns how to distinguish the breathing sounds that indicate pulmonary oedema from those suggest-ing pneumonia. Rules of treatment can now refer to the presence or absence of such sounds (Dreyfus & Dreyfus, 1986).

In stable situations, advanced beginners feel secure with practice directed by orders, rules and procedures, or common practice. In unstable situations, they lack the flexibility and clinical knowledge to adapt to rapidly changing situations. Their responsibility does not often include determining what to do, or even how to do it, but involves following what has been designed and structured by others. Because the demands of clinical situations often outstrip beginners' clinical judgements, they 'delegate up' their observations and concerns and rely on the judgements of more experienced clinicians who surround them (Benner *et al.*, 1992).

The novice and advanced beginner recognise learned components and then apply learned rules and procedures. They have little, if any, sense of responsibility for the outcomes of their acts. Assuming that they have not made any mistakes, an unfortunate outcome is viewed as the result of inadequately specified elements or rules.

## Stage 3: Competence

With more experience, the individual is faced with a sense of 'what is important', rather than focusing on context-free and situational elements, in the real world. The competent nurse will no longer automatically go from patient to patient in a prescribed order, but will assess the urgency of their needs and plan work accordingly. The plan is based on considerable conscious, abstract, analytic contemplation of the problem (Dreyfus & Dreyfus, 1986).

The competent performer feels responsible for, and thus is emotionally involved in, the product of his/her choice. Competence is typified by the nurse who has been on the job in the same or similar situations for 2 or 3 years (Benner, 1984). While the nurse understands and decides in a detached manner, he/she becomes intensely involved in what occurs thereafter. An outcome that is successful is deeply satisfying and leaves a vivid memory of both the chosen plan and of the situation itself. Disasters likewise are not easily forgotten (Dreyfus & Dreyfus, 1986).

## Stage 4: Proficiency

Up to this point the learner of a new skill has made his/her choices consciously after contemplating various choices. The proficient performer intuitively and non-consciously organises and understands his/her task; detached choice and deliberation are rare (Dreyfus & Dreyfus, 1986). Performance is guided by maxims: cryptic instructions passed on by experts that make sense only if the performer has a deep understanding of the situation (Polanyi, 1958). The perspective is not thought out, but presents itself. Both proficient and expert skills are characterised by rapid, fluid behaviour that bears no similarity to the slow, detached reasoning of the problem-solving process. Memories of similar situations, experienced previously, trigger plans similar to those that worked in the past. The proficient nurse learns, from experience, what events to expect in a particular situation, to recognise when the expected normal picture does not materialise, and how to modify plans in response to those events. Proficient performance can usually be found in nurses who have worked with similar patient populations for approximately 3–5 years (Benner, 1984).

**Stage 5: Expert**
The expert performer no longer relies on analytic principles to connect her or his understanding of the situation to an appropriate action. An expert generally knows what to do based on mature and practised understanding. Capability for the routine is essential for competence, but it is the handling of non-routine matters, which defines the expert (Eraut, 1994). The expert nurse is totally engaged in skilful performance. 'When things are proceeding normally, experts don't solve problems and don't make decisions, they do what normally works' (Dreyfus & Dreyfus, 1986, pp. 30–31). Capturing the descriptions of expert performance is difficult because the nurse operates from a deep understanding of the total situation (Benner, 1984; Dreyfus and Dreyfus, 1986).

The model holds that in learning, changes in four general aspects of performance are reflected:

(1) Movement from a reliance on abstract principles and rules to use of past, concrete experience.
(2) A shift from a reliance on analytic rule-based thinking to intuition. Many nurses attribute some of their decision-making to intuition, and see it as a valid part of their practice. Others do not view intuition as 'legitimate knowledge'. Benner (1984) defines intuition as 'understanding without rationale'. Her view is criticised by some who believe that 'intuition involves the use of a sound rational, relevant knowledge base in situations that, through experience, are so familiar that the person has learned to recognise and act on appropriate patterns in the presenting problem' (Easen & Wilcockson, 1996, p. 672).
(3) Change in the nurse's perception of the situation from one in which it is viewed as a compilation of equally relevant parts, to an increasingly complex whole, in which certain parts are relevant.
(4) Passage from a detached observer, standing outside the situation, to one of a position of involvement, fully engaged in the situation (Benner *et al.*, 1992).

Novices, for example, may not recognise the relationship(s) between cues and states of health. As a result, the novice tends to believe that if a cue is present there is a 100% chance of a particular state of health, e.g. anuria in a catheterised patient is attributed to hypovolaemia, rather than a catheter blockage. Experienced practitioners not only have greater knowledge for decision making, they have also developed knowledge structures that enable them to identify more cues and to make better use of these during decision making about patient care.

---

**Activity**

Think of the development of your practice and decision making.

* Is your development adequately represented by Benner's five-stage model of skill acquisition?
* Have other things influenced your development?
* Some authors criticise the model because it assumes that nurses always learn from experience, do you think learning always happens?

---

## Reflective practice

One concept that has been widely embraced throughout the nursing community in raising awareness of the knowledge that underpins nursing practice is that of reflective practice. Two conceptions of reflection are evident in the literature. The first, which will be discussed here, views it as a theory of practice (Schon, 1983a, 1987), the second, which is discussed in Chapter 10, views reflection as an element of experiential learning (Kolb, 1984).

The knowledge embedded in clinical practice can be made explicit through reflection. There are many theoretical accounts of reflection in the literature. Boyd & Fales (1983) describe reflection as 'the process of internally examining and explaining an issue of concern triggered by an experience, which creates and clarifies meanings in terms of self and which results in a changed perceptual perspective'. Johns (2000) suggests that reflection is a window through which practitioners can view and focus their 'self' within the context of their own lived experiences in ways that enable them to confront, understand and work towards resolving the contradictions within practice between what is desirable and actual practice. Reflection has been influential in uncovering the knowledge and intuition that underpin nursing practice, as well as providing insight into the transformation of knowing-in-action into knowledge-in-action.

While the literature includes a variety theories and guidance about the process of reflection (for examples of these, see Schon, 1987; Johns, 2000), the differences appear to be, largely, those of terminology. In a review of Schon's work, Harbison (1991) defined the reflective practitioner as: 'one who constantly "watches" herself in action: discovers and acknowledges the limits of her expertise, attempts to extend this . . . she is professionally mature enough to reveal uncertainty, and accept the risks inherent in all decision making' (Harbison, 1991, p. 404).

With the belief that the process of reflection should incorporate the practitioner's experiences (feeling and thoughts) as well as best evidence, Atkins & Murphy (1993) describe three reflective stages:

(1) An awareness of uncomfortable feelings and thoughts about situations and people.
(2) An examination of knowledge, including critical thought and best evidence.
(3) Perspective transformation: the ultimate goal of reflection where learning and practice change occurs.

An 'examination of knowledge' enables analysis of best evidence, the 'examination of uncomfortable feelings and thoughts' is likely to elucidate the experience of the practitioners and to uncover some of the hidden knowledge applied in practice. In combination, the two provide detailed information about the knowledge that informs clinical practice. The final stage, perspective transformation, enables the benefits of any learning from this process to be acted upon, changed and implemented as appropriate.

---

**Activity**

Think about the way that you learn in clinical practice. Think about a particular skill or task that you have learnt recently, and about how you learnt to carry it out; for example taking blood, or administering intravenous fluid.

- Did you learn in the way described by Benner in consecutive stages?
- Did you learn by reflecting on your practice?

Think about how you or others make changes to clinical practice, and about a recent change to your practice.

- How was the need for the change identified?

---

Reflection recognises the central role that experiential learning plays in the development of competence and also emphasises the individual's responsibility to maintain and increase the level of that competence (Schon, 1983b; Benner, 1984). The recognition of the limits of one's own competence is vital if new roles assumed by nurses are to be successful. Failure to do so can be devastating to the nurse and to others concerned (see Chapters 10 and 14 for more information about adverse events).

While scope of practice and professional standards are determined to some extent by an individual's employing organisation, doctors and nurses are also regulated by professional bodies. All healthcare professionals operate within some sort of establishment that places limitations or boundaries on their practice. In terms of official allocation of responsibility by the medical and nursing professions, both address the issue through codes of conduct, the principle function of which is to provide a point of reference upon which professional practice may be based.

# Professional regulation

With the current and ongoing changes to roles and role boundaries, there has been a concurrent and necessary change in the culture of health care in which more equal relationships and collaborative working is becoming the norm. The complexity of modern care is such that no single profession can reasonably assume accountability or responsibility for all care. The current lack of clarity about responsibilities are a cause for concern. Arguably however, the situation may change as it is being addressed through the development of the NHS's 'Regulation in the Health Professions' (Department of Health, 2001, 2004), and through the Council for Healthcare Regulatory Excellence (CHRE) established in 2003, which promotes best practice and consistency in the regulation of healthcare professionals.

Regulation ensures standards of practice and protects the public as far as possible against the risk of poor practice by regulated practitioners. It works by setting agreed standards of practice and competence, by registering those who are competent to practice and (if statutory) restricting the use of specified titles to those who are registered; and by applying sanctions such as removing from the register any whose fitness to practise is impaired (Department of Health, 2004).

## *The Nursing and Midwifery Council and regulation*

As well as issuing details of the scope of practice, the NMC holds a register of those nurses and midwives who meet the minimum standards for registration. It also has the power to decide whether to remove an individual from the register for misconduct, lack of competence or ill health. The overriding objective of the NMC is to safeguard the health and well-being of persons using or needing the services of registrants; that is, it protects patients. Public protection is key. The NMC's role is not to promote the status of the professions or to provide legal advice; that is the function of professional bodies such as the Royal College of Nursing.

## Responsibility for care

Health care has moved towards an approach to patient care that challenges traditional role boundaries. The current situation reflects the expectations of The Heathrow Debate (Department of Health, 1994), which indicated that amongst other things, the drivers for change in health care would lead to a reallocation of tasks between nurses and other healthcare professionals.

### Between doctors and nurses

As previously indicated, nurses are taking on roles traditionally assumed by medical staff and are, simultaneously, taking on new and increasing responsibility for patient care and outcomes. However, according to the General Medical Council (GMC) (1995), medicine's governing body in the UK, ultimate responsibility for patient care still rests with the medical profession. As a result, while their contribution to patient care is increasingly being recognised, nurses are still often powerless other than to give advice about patient management, rather than to order it.

Interestingly, the latest statement from the GMC with regard to the allocation of work to non-medical staff was published in 1995. It is, arguably, out of date given recent changes within health care. *Good Medical Practice* (General Medical Council, 1995, p. 3) states:

> *You may delegate medical care to nurses and other health care staff who are not registered medical practitioners if you believe it is best for the patient. But you must be sure that the person to whom you delegate is competent to undertake the procedure or therapy involved. When delegating care or treatment, you must always pass on enough information about the patient and the treatment needed. You will still be responsible for managing the patient's care.*

The situation may change, as it is being addressed through the development of the NHS's *Modernising Regulation in the Health Professions* (Department of Health, 2001), currently a consultation document. The GMC admits within the document that its 'accountability is largely implicit . . . (and) . . . that this is unsatisfactory for a modern regulatory body carrying this level of responsibility and public trust'.

---

**Activity**

Think about how the delivery of care is organised in your place of work, and in those of your friends or colleagues.

* Do you know what your responsibility is in the delivery of care?

---

### Between nurses and healthcare assistants

In nursing, changes to roles and role boundaries have resulted in the delegation of 'nursing care' to healthcare assistants (HCAs) and other unregistered health workers. The expanding role of this unregulated group of staff has been widely debated. The literature suggests that they work in a number of settings and carry out a range of tasks, and that the scope of their role is affected by the patient population and the methods of delegation employed by registered nurses (RNs) (Warr, 2002; Hancock *et al.*, 2005). The reaction of RNs to others taking on fundamental nursing roles, appears to be, in part, a mixture of relief at getting help in a time of critical staff shortages (McKenna, 1995; Francomb, 1997; Rolfe *et al.*, 1999; McKenna & Hasson, 2002), unease at giving ground on traditional areas of work (Hurst & Ball, 1990; Ormandy *et al.*, 2001; O'Dowd, 2002), and concern about the dilution of skill mix associated with it (Thornley, 2000).

The restructuring of roles between registered nurses and HCAs is a challenging part of the new ways of working in health care. The move demands new ways of thinking about the nursing role and care delivery. While a difficult transition the real issue is not one of a divided approach but one of unity in the provision of quality patient care. This view will be easier to adopt once the regulation of this group has been addressed.

In *The NHS Plan* (Department of Health, 2000), the government promised to publish proposals for the regulation of support workers, and 2004 saw the publication of a consultation document: *Regulation of Health Care Staff in England and Wales* (Department of Health, 2004). Within the document are three main reasons for regulating healthcare support staff:

(1) To protect the public by requiring these staff to meet standards of practice, conduct and training, and by dealing with those who do not meet the standards.
(2) To provide a regulated workforce of practitioners who can safely fill jobs vacated by professional practitioners as they take on extended medical roles, and who can build on this to go on to professional practice if they wish.

(3)  To plug gaps in the overall regulatory framework so that all staff in health and social care whose work could impact on patients or clients are subject to similar regulation.

It is anticipated that, following the results of this consultation, statutory regulation could be put in place for assistants and support staff by the end of 2007 (Department of Health, 2004).

# The future

The advancement of the nursing role in health care and the unprecedented changes in care delivery, with role expansion, are clearly evident in practice. In the UK new roles such as nurse consultants, matrons and clinical nurse practitioners have been introduced to effect these changes, which are discussed in Chapter 13. The result has been that a considerable amount of health care is now provided by these and other RNs, practising interdependently, managing case loads of patients and clients in a variety of hospital and community settings.

## *Beyond initial RN registration*

As part of the development and extension of the roles of registered nurses, the NMC in the UK released a consultation document relating to proposals to establish a framework for a standard for a level of nursing practice beyond initial registration (Nursing and Midwifery Council, 2005). As with the majority of the work of the NMC, the purpose of these proposals is to protect the public by setting a standard for any nurse who is working at this level. It will also clarify the level of care the public can expect from the new and numerous nursing roles that have been established (e.g. nurse consultant, nurse practitioner). Plans for such regulation are not unique, as the GMC released a specialist register in 1995 to regulate the standard of medical practice of consultants.

At the time of writing this book, the NMC is proposing to establish a sub-part register for nurses who achieve an advanced level of practice. It states that the characteristics of nurses who are working at this level of practice are that they work both independently and interdependently (Nursing and Midwifery Council, 2005), by:

• taking responsibility for case management
• making differential diagnoses
• planning and providing care and treatment, including prescribing medication, in collaboration with others as appropriate
• providing health education, counselling and leadership.

They state (Nursing and Midwifery Council, 2005, p. 8) that those eligible will be:

*A registered nurse who has command of an expert knowledge base and clinical competence, is able to make complex clinical decisions using expert clinical judgement, is an essential member of an interdependent health care team and whose role is determined by the context in which s/he practices.*

Following the consultation and consideration of the report by Council, and approval by the Privy Council, plans for the post-registration nursing framework will be established, with implementation no later than September 2010.

## Summary

- Nursing as a profession has developed considerably since its origins in the 1800s.
- Nursing has been transformed from a gender-determined vocation to a current-day profession with its own unique and increasing contribution to health and patient care.
- The Novice to Expert Model and reflective practice help to explain how nurses develop their professional and practical knowledge.
- Changes to the roles and remit of professional nursing practice have occurred as a result of a number of factors, which include patient needs and service requirements.
- The ongoing development of the nursing profession has heightened the need for professional regulation, which aims to ensure that nurses understand and accept the responsibilities inherent in providing patient care.
- The blurring of boundaries between nurses, doctors and healthcare assistants has increased the need to clarify ultimate responsibility for patient care.
- A new framework for post-registration nurses, to enable competent individuals to make complex clinical decisions, is being developed by the NMC.

# References

Atkins, S & Murphy, K (1993) Reflection: a review of the literature. *Journal of Advanced Nursing* 18: 1118–92.

Benner, P (1984) *From Novice to Expert: Excellence and Power in Clinical Nursing Practice*. Addison Wesley, Menlo Park, California.

Benner, P, Tanner, C & Chelsea, C (1992) From beginner to expert gaining a differentiated clinical world in critical care nursing. *Advances in Nursing Science* 14 (3): 13–28.

Boyd, E & Fales, A (1983) Reflective learning: Key to learning from experience. *Journal of Humanistic Psychology* 23 (2): 99–117.

Buchan, J (2002) Global nursing shortages are often a symptom of wider health system or societal ailments. *British Medical Journal* 324: 751–2.

Davies, C (1995) *Gender and the Professional Predicament in Nursing*. Open University Press, Buckingham.

Department of Health (1994) *The Challenges for Nursing and Midwifery in the 21st Century: A Report of the Heathrow Debate Between Chief Nursing Officers of England, Wales, Scotland and Northern Ireland*. HMSO, London.

Department of Health (2000) *The NHS Plan: A Plan for Investment, A Plan for Reform*. HMSO, London.

Department of Health (2001) *Modernising Regulation in the Health Professions*. The Stationery Office, London.

Department of Health (2004) *Consultation Document: Regulation of Health Care Staff in England and Wales*. HMSO, London.

Doering, L (1992) Power and knowledge in nursing: a feminist post structuralist view. *Advances In Nursing Science* 14: 24–33.

Dreyfus, H & Dreyfus, S (1980) A five stage model of the mental activities involved in directed skill acquisition. Unpublished study, University of California, Berkeley.

Dreyfus, H & Dreyfus, S (1986) *Mind Over Machine: The Power of Human Intuition and Expertise in the Era of the Computer*. The Free Press, New York.

Dreyfus, S (1982) Formal models V's human situational understanding: inherent limitations on modelling of business expertise. *Office Technology and People* 1: 133–55.

Easen, P & Wilcockson, J (1996) Intuition and rational decision making in professional thinking: a false dichotomy? *Journal of Advanced Nursing* 24: 667–73.

Eraut, M (1994) *Developing Professional Knowledge and Competence*. Falmer Press, London.

Francomb, H (1997) Do we need support workers in the maternity services? *British Journal of Midwifery* 5 (11): 672–6.

General Medical Council (1995) *Good Medical Practice: Duties of a Doctor, Guidance from the General Medical Council*. GMC, London.

Hancock, H, Campbell, S, Ramproguus, V & Kilgour, J (2005) Role development in health care assistants: the impact of education on practice. *Journal of Evaluation in Clinical Practice* 11 (5): 489–98.

Harbison, J (1991) Clinical decision making in nursing. *Journal of Advanced Nursing* 16: 404–407.

Harding, C & Grieg, M (1994) Issues of accountability in the assessment of practice. *Nurse Education Today* 14 (2): 118–23.

Henderson, V (1969) *The Nature of Nursing*. Macmillan, New York.

Higgins, A (2003) The developing role of the consultant. *Nursing Management* 10 (1): 22–8.

Holden, R J (1991) Responsibility and autonomous nursing practice. *Journal of Advanced Nursing* 16 (4): 398–403.

Hurst, K & Ball, J (1990) A tailor made workforce for 2000. *Nursing Standard* 4: 35–6.

Johns, C C (2000) *Becoming a Reflective Practitioner*. Blackwell Science, Oxford.

Kolb, D A (1984) *Experiential Learning: Experience as the Source of Learning and Development*. Prentice Hall. USA.

McKenna, H (1995) Nursing skill mix substitutions and quality of care: an exploration of assumptions from the research literature. *Journal of Advanced Nursing* 21: 452–9.

McKenna, H & Hasson, F (2002) A study of skill mix issues in midwifery: a multi-method approach. *Journal of Advanced Nursing* 31 (1): 52–61.

Nightingale, F (1865) *Rules for Admission and Training Nurses at St Thomas's Hospital*. London.

Nursing and Midwifery Council (2002) *Code of Professional Conduct*. NMC, London.

Nursing and Midwifery Council (2005) *Consultation on a Framework for the Standard for Post-registration Nursing*. NMC, London.

O'Dowd, A (2002) DH banks on invisible workforce of 37,000 staff. *Nursing Times* 98: 10–11.

Ormandy, P, Long, A, Johnson, M & Hulme, C (2001) *Evaluation of Workforce Development in Critical Care Interim Report (2)*. Health Care Practice Research and Development Unit, Salford University.

Peterson, M J (1978) *The Medical Profession In Mid-Victorian London*. University of California Press, Los Angeles, USA.

Polanyi, M (1958) *Personal Knowledge: Towards A Post Critical Philosophy*. Routledge and Kegan Paul, London.

Rogers, M (1970) *An Introduction to the Theoretical Basis of Nursing*. F A Davis, Philadelphia.

Rolfe, G, Jackson, N, Gardner, L, Jasper, M & Gale, A (1999) Developing the role of the generic healthcare support worker: phase 1 of an action research study. *International Journal of Nursing Studies* 36: 323–34.

Schon, D A (1983a) *The Reflective Practitioner: How Professionals Think In Action*. Temple Smith, London.

Schon, D A (1983b) From technical rationality to reflection in action. In Dowie, J & Elstein, A (eds) *Professional Judgement: A Reader In Clinical Decision Making*. Cambridge University Press, Cambridge.

Schon, D A (1987) *Educating the Reflective Practitioner*. Jossey Bass, San Francisco.

Statutory Instrument (2002) *The Nursing and Midwifery Order* (SI no. 253). The Stationery Office, Norwich.

Thompson, W (1906) The overtrained nurse. *New York Medical Journal* 83: 845–9.

Thornley, C (2000) A question of competence? Re-evaluating the roles of the nursing auxiliary and health care assistants in the NHS. *Journal of Clinical Nursing* 9: 451–8.

Warr, J (2002) Experiences and perceptions of newly prepared HCAs. *Nurse Education Today* 22: 241–50.

# Index